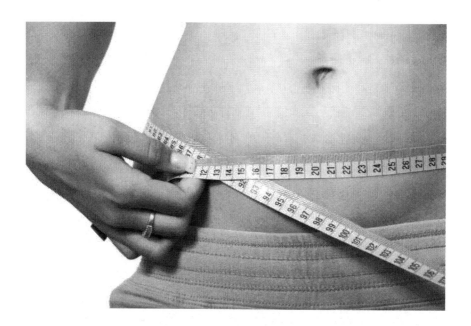

*By Emily Lewis*

# The guide to intermittent fasting for beginners

# A Combination Of Keto Diet And Intermittent Fasting In Meal Plans On A Budget To Help You Boost Metabolism, Heal Your Body, Lose Weight & Gain Muscle

# Table of content

# Chapter One

# Introduction

Intermittent fasting (IF) is presently the leading global health, wellness and fitness trend. People all over the world are using this method to lose weight, gain health benefits and simplify their lifestyles.

Before going into details of intermittent fasting it's important to understand that it not one of the fad diets that claim to *"melt your fat away"* or *"lose 10 pounds in 10 days"*, rather it's a lifestyle change that you can maintain for a long period with minimal deviation. Moreover, there is scientific research that prove that it has significant effects on your physical and mental health and may even help you live longer.

## INTERMITTENT FASTING: WHAT IS IT?

According to Cambridge English dictionary intermittent

means something that does not occur continuously, while fasting means abstaining from eating or going without food. Thus, intermittent fasting (IF) is not diet, rather it's a cyclical eating pattern that has phases of fasting and eating. It is not about what you eat it's more about when you eat. It's a strategy to schedule your meals in a way that you get the most out of them.

Most of the intermittent fasting methods does not specify the foods that you need to consume but focus on when to eat them. However, during your eating period, there are foods items that will help you multiply the benefits of Intermittent fasting, but we will discuss it in later sections of the book.

## DOES THIS EATING PATTERN REALLY HELP?

Yes, in many ways. Most noticeably, it will help you lose those extra pounds and get lean without going on a crazy diet or cutting your calories to bare minimum. On the contrary, most of the people can even eat the same amount of calories they were eating before but in a designated span of period. Additionally, intermittent fasting is a great method to lose fat without losing muscle mass, at the same time it requires minimal behavior change. Hence IF falls in the category of health and fitness interventions that are simple enough to implement and significant enough in making an actual difference

## HOW DOES INTERMITTENT FASTING WORK?

Some of you might be skeptical that how can we lose fat

eating the same food only by changing the eating pattern? To understand this first we need to understand the terms'; "the fasted state" and "the fed state" and the difference between the two.

The fed state is when our body is digesting and absorbing food that we consume. Normally, the body goes into fed state as soon as you start eating and it lasts for five to six hours as you digest the food you just ate and the nutrients are absorbed in the body. During the fed state, it is near to impossible for your body to burn any fat as your insulin levels are high.

Once your body is done processing the meal it goes in to the post –absorptive state that remains for about 8 to 10 hours and after that your body is ready to enter the fasted state. In the fasted state your insulin levels become low and your body starts burning fat that was inaccessible during the fed state.

But do we really wait for 10-12 hours after our meal to actually let our body go into fasted state and start burning fat? In our typical eating patterns that rarely happens but people who adopt intermittent fasting do it and that's why they start losing fat even without changing what they eat, how much they eat, or how often they exercise. Fasting places your body in a fat burning state that you rarely make it to during a usual eating timetable.

## WHY INSULIN LEVELS ARE SO IMPORTANT?

What is most striking thing about what we eat nowadays? Open your refrigerator and take a look inside, or on the dining table in front of you, or the tables of people dining around you in a restaurant, you would see soft –drinks, breads, chips, bakery items, confectioneries, the vitamin rich sugar water...and the list is on and on but you must be able to appreciate that the common thing amongst them is that all have something unnatural about them.

We need not be nutrition or health expert to know that foods are not created in this way by nature to be consumed neither are we programmed to consume food in this form.

These are changes made in present times, foods scientifically designed and crafted to make it extremely palatable for the taste buds, irrespective of the damage it causes to the body.

When you eat food, it causes the blood sugar to rise. In response pancreas secretes a hormone called "Insulin", to drive the extra sugar into cells. The insulin receptors in cells containing glucose have to be clear for the proper action of the hormone. If this process is not working properly, insulin resistance develops and as glucose is not able to enter cells, it stays in the blood. Now as the cells are not getting the fuel and energy for their function, they keep signaling to the brain for more release of insulin, resulting in sugar cravings. These persistent increased blood glucose levels also contribute in increased risk for many diseases such as type 2 diabetes and hyperlipidemias (increased blood fats).

Foods rich in starch and sugar increase your hunger and sugar cravings and avoiding them keeps it at an adequate level.

As we talk about hunger, we have to differentiate between Unhealthy or damaging hunger and the normal hunger.

The damaging hunger comes at a blood sugar which is not low enough for normal hunger, indulges you in over eating, and increases the drive to eat much more calories that you actually require. The combination of this damaging hunger followed by over eating leads to diabetes and other health issues like high LDL levels and heart problems.

On the other hand actual or normal hunger appears only after your body has consumed much of the calories from the previous meal and your blood sugar level has reached a certain level and thus requires re-energizing. The problem of damaging hunger is also brought on by the wrong choice of food. Highly processed foods and foods with high glycemic index and simple carbohydrates cause addiction in our bodies, thus the symptoms that we experience after few hours of consuming these foods are actually the withdrawal symptoms mistaken as hunger. The result is a vicious cycle of eating-feeling withdrawal symptoms-eating again, the symptoms get relieved initially by eating, but the symptoms reappear again after few hours. To break this vicious cycle you don't need to eat every time you feel damaging hunger, but the correct response is that you choose when to eat which stops this false or damaging hunger. With good alteration of diet, damaging hunger slowly reduces and is resolved, letting people to feel satisfied with less eating. As said at the start, trying to limit or count the calories is an ineffective way for controlling false hunger. You need not to limit calories, but to desire fewer calories..

# Chapter Two

# The scientific evidence regarding intermittent fasting and weight loss

Human body stores energy in form of fats. Typically when we eat any food, our digestive system breaks down it into glucose, which is the simplest form of sugar that enters the bloodstream. In response to raised blood sugar levels, a hormone called Insulin is secreted by Pancreas, to drive the extra sugar into cells and use it for energy.

As glucose is the simplest and easiest molecule for our body to convert and use as energy, it is the preferred form of energy source. By choosing glucose as the energy source, the fats are usually not needed and remain stored. But when we are fasting and not eating anything our body makes many changes to make the other source of energy i.e. fats, more accessible for us. The changes are both hormonal as well as in the nervous system.

The hormones mostly involved in this mechanism are:

1. **Insulin:** As already discussed insulin increases when we eat, and it lowers significantly when we fast. Low levels of insulin facilitates burning fat for energy requirements of our body.

2. **Human growth hormone (HGH):** This is the hormone that helps in building muscle mass and losing fat. During fasting state the levels of this hormone really spike to almost 5 times than when you are eating.

3. **Norepinephrine (noradrenaline):** Noradrenaline (norepinephrine) is a hormone and a neurotransmitter produced by our brain and sympathetic nerves in reaction to some stimuli to cope with certain situations known as -fight-or- flight response. During fasting, your nervous system sends norepinephrine to your fat cells to stimulate them to break down into three fatty acids that can be utilized for energy requirements of the body. These changes in the hormones during a short –term fast may help your metabolism to increase by 3.6–14%.

People in general and especially those who are weight-conscious, or trying to lose weight, are usually aware of the term 'calories' written as "Kcal" in the nutrient details of many food products and recipes. A calorie is a unit that measures energy. These are usually used to calculate the amount of energy contained in various foods and beverages. The relationship of calories with weight loss can be described in most simple words as you need to eat less calories than your body burns each day in order to lose weight, in other you need to be calorie deficient. Although, the focus in intermittent fasting is not to count calories, however, the magnificence of this method is that you automatically end up eating less calories by adopting intermittent fasting life style.

Therefore the key to success is that you take advantage of the increased metabolism and control your calories intake to reap maximum benefits of intermittent fasting. Binge eating and eating very large meals during the eating window may stop you from fully enjoying the weight loss and other good effects of intermittent fasting.

Research Studies have shown that intermittent fasting is a very powerful weight loss tool.

An in-depth review in 2014, comparing the Intermittent fasting vs. daily calorie restriction for type 2 diabetes prevention, found that intermittent fasting was able to achieve 3-8% weight loss in 3- 24 weeks, which was significantly higher than the amount of weight loss by calories restriction.

In the same study, it was also observed that participants experienced about 4-7% reduction in their waist circumference, it denotes that they lost their belly fat which is the most dangerous type of fat as it builds up around vital organs and is the biggest risk factor for many diseases including high blood pressure and heart diseases.

In another systematic review, it was found that intermittent fasting causes less muscle loss than the more standard method of continuous calorie restriction.

# OTHER BENEFITS OF INTERMITTENT FASTING

Weight loss is great, but the benefits of intermittent fasting does not stop there. Other benefits of intermittent fasting are:

- Intermittent fasting simplifies your life style

One commodity that we all are always short of is TIME. Talking specifically about diet and eating, many diet plans that look marvelous on paper are complete failures when it comes to actually implementing them, because the time required to prepare those meals most often becomes the biggest hurdle in following the diet. Intermittent fasting is all about changing behavior with simplifying your life and reducing stress. How good it is that you can just start your day with a glass of water or a cup of coffee and work for another 5-6 hours without worrying for your food. Even for people who do not mind cooking and cooking three meals a day is not a hassle for them, a life style that requires only two meals translates into planning one less meal, cooking one less meal and thus stressing less about one meal. It makes life quite simpler and most people like that.

- You may live longer on intermittent fasting

People around that world have believed that restricting food intake is related to longevity, the basis of this belief is when you are starving; your body finds ways to extend your life. Scientists also shared the same belief and that started their further inquest in this matter However, people want to enjoy their life and starving themselves in order to live longer is not a pleasing idea for many of us.

The first scientific study that made breakthrough in this field was way back in 1946, which showed that intermittent fasting extended life in mice. This discovery brought with itself the good news that intermittent fasting is able to activate many of the same mechanisms for extending life as with restricting calorie intake for a long duration (or starvation). Afterwards many human studies were also done that agreed that you can get the benefit of longevity from intermittent fasting without the hassle of undergoing starvation. The studies have also shown that there are changes in gene expression related to longevity and protection against disease.

- Intermittent fasting controls inflammation

Inflammation is a common factor present in patients suffering from heart disease and stroke and considered as a sign of athrogenic response to the damage by various stimuli. Based on the knowledge and scientific evidence we have now, it is extremely important to control the risk factors that result in increased inflammatory response in the body. These risk factors are mainly smoking, high blood pressure and LDL (bad cholesterol). There are studies that show that adoption of intermittent fasting is directly associated with decrease in various biomarkers of inflammation.

- Intermittent fasting improves heart health

Heart attacks and strokes are caused by atherosclerotic plaques formation and high levels of triglycerides in the body, these plaques under unfavorable conditions release contents which when come in contact with blood results in clot formation. This clot can get detached from the arterial walls and cause blockage in heart arteries causing heart attack or brain arteries causing hemorrhagic stroke. Research has shown Intermittent fasting may reduce the threat of heart diseases by reducing its risk factors including "bad" LDL cholesterol, blood triglycerides, inflammatory markers, blood sugar and insulin resistance

- Intermittent fasting improves brain health

Latest research has shown that when brain cell metabolism is shifted away from sugar in favor of burning fats, it not only prevents neurodegenerative conditions such as Alzheimer's but also actually helps in treatment of diseases like Alzheimer's disease, Parkinson's disease, and epilepsy.

In addition, intermittent fasting also increases the level of the brain hormone BDNF, which may help in the growth of new nerve cells.

*Chapter Three*

# History of fasting

F asting has been associated with treatment of many health conditions for more than two thousand years. Hippocrates of Cos (c 460 – c370 BC) is considered the father of modern medicine. In the Hippocratic collection, fasting is the only measure recorded as the treatment of many health conditions including epilepsy. Hippocrates in one of his scriptures wrote, "To eat when you are sick, is to feed your illness".

Five centuries later, in Biblical times also, fasting was documented as treatment of epilepsy. Later, other Greek thinkers and writers including Plutarch, Plato and Aristotle also reverberated the same sentiments about fasting. Plutarch stated, "Instead of using medicine, better fast today". These ancient Greek thinkers believed that best medical treatment can be understood by observing nature. It is common among both animals and humans that they stop eating when they are sick. It is the natural doctor within oneself. This feeling is common to everybody. Consider the last time, you were down with a sickness such as common cold, you might remember that you did not want to eat at all. This is the nature's healing mechanism. Ancient Indian healers believed in giving rest to the gut when suffering from diarrhea or indigestion. The practice is still prevalent in the India and other Asian countries.

Thus fasting is deep-rooted into human tradition, and is as old as mankind itself.

The ancient philosophers also believed in the significant effect of fasting in improving cognition. You can relate to it, remember the large time you had a large feast like on Thanksgiving. How did you feel afterwards? Alert and energetic or sluggish and sleepy? Most probably the latter and there is a scientific reason for it; when we consume a large meal, the focus of all blood circulation becomes the digestive tract; to digest that big meal, and this is done at the expense of diverting blood circulation from your brain, therefore limiting your cognitive abilities and feeling sleepy also known as food coma.. More so, you will understand better; consider the office hours after lunch break especially if there is any celebration in the office. Working after eating lunch becomes a real challenge, isn't it?

In modern history, one of the great proponents of fasting include Philip Paracelsus, who is the founder of Modern western medicine and toxicology. In one of his books he wrote; "Fasting is the greatest remedy – the physician within". Benjamin Franklin; one of the United States of America's founding fathers and the leading author, scientist and political theorist, once suggested that resting and fasting are the best of all medicines.

Another important aspect of fasting is fasting for religious or spiritual reasons and this has remained practice of almost every major religion or faith in the world. Christianity, Judaism and Islam share a common belief in the spiritual and healing powers of fasting. Although, implemented on the physical body, it is considered as the tool for spiritual purification and cleansing alongside many physical and mental benefits.

Muslims observe mandatory fasting in the holy month of Ramadan, from sunrise to sunset for 29 or 30 days depending upon the sighting of the moon. Additionally, they are also encouraged to fast on every Monday and Thursday and three days; 13th, 14th, 15th of the lunar month. Research related to fating has for the most part remained focused on Ramadan fasting. This fasting is different from other fasting rituals as fluids are also prohibited during fasting hours. The studies found that fasting Muslims also have some degree of dehydration in them. More interestingly, it was found that since it is allowed to eat between sunset and sunrise, the number of calories consumed during this period actually rises considerably during the fasting month. Devouring large meals at time of breaking fast (Aftar) and keeping fast (Sahoor) actually take some of the benefits away from the fasting regime.

Amongst other religions, in Buddhism food is only eaten in the mornings and then the followers fast from noon till the next morning. Additionally there are water-fasts only for days or even weeks on end. Greek orthodox Christians have also been documented to fast for almost 180-200 days in a year. Crete is a beautiful island in Greece, a favorite tourist destination, various nutrition and wellness writers have depicted Crete as a classical picture of the healthy Mediterranean diet. But the fact that most of these writers tend to over-look is that majority of people in Crete follow the Greek traditional fasting method.

So, fasting is truthfully a practice that has endured the test of time. Most of the learned men ever lived on our planet have agreed that fasting is beneficial for health. In more than 1000 years of written history, if there were any adverse effects of fasting, they must be out in the limelight by now. Hence, we can follow the variants of classical fating- the intermittent fasting- with confidence.

## RENAISSANCE OF FASTING - INTERMITTENT FASTING

In modern history, in the year 1921, researcher, Woodyatt made two ground breaking observations, first that two compounds acetones and beta-hydroxybutyric acid (ketones) appear in a normal person after fasting and secondly that same compounds appear in persons using a diet containing high proportion of fats and very low proportion of carbohydrates. At the same time, another researcher Dr Wilder in Mayo Clinic also suggested that the benefits of fasting can be obtained if ketosis can be achieved by use of high fat, low carb diet. He also proposed that keto diet can be used safely for longer periods in patients with epilepsy.

Since then experts have been studying the effect of fasting and the linkage of fasting and keto diet for treatment of epilepsy, for weight loss, for preventing diabetes, heart disease and other metabolic disorders.

Intermittent fasting as an approach for weight loss has

been around for many years, but a renewed interest was ignited when a BBC broadcast journalist Dr. Michael Mosley, in 2012, produced a TV documentary by the name *Eat Fast, Live Longer* and also wrote a book *The Fast Diet* . The trend resonated well with other media personalities and soon journalist Kate Harrison came out with her book The *5:2 Diet* based on her personal experience.

The intermittent fasting produced a firm positive buzz all around and anecdotes of its effectiveness circulated and impressed all and sundry.

Other than media personalities, doctors and other scientific researchers also pitched in and produced various evidence-based resources using scientific research and their clinical experience along with nutritional and socioeconomic considerations illustrating why we become fat and how we can use intermittent fasting to get rid of this excess weight in the most simple and doable way i.e. intermittent fasting.


## HUMAN FOOD CHOICES OVER THE YEARS

It is a well –known fact that overweight and obesity is the "epidemic" of modern times, it not only have physical ,psychological and social implications, but is considered a major health issue contributing to development of serious medical conditions including heart disease, stroke, type 2 diabetes and certain types of cancers e.g. colorectal cancer. It is also associated with several other conditions like , osteoarthritis, liver disease, snoring, sleep apnea, depression and GERD(Gastro-esophageal reflux disease), also commonly known as Acid Reflux disease.

Modern biomedical science has made leaps of advancement in technology in the last 50 years or so, but conventional medicine has failed to control the occurrence of these top killer diseases, i.e. cancer and heart disease.

As a result of the continuous drumming of" low fat, high carb" as standard dietary advice by dietary associations and experts since many years, people have been thriving on a typical diet full of sugars, carbohydrates and processed foods with omega 6 oils.

However, we don't need to tell you that this typical high-carb diet is a failure. Just look at the people around us. Large size people with big bellies are everywhere and obesity rates are soaring in all age groups even children. We try to limit the fat that we eat, as much as possible, and yet we gain weight.

While the high Carb, processed foods high in sugar and salt consumed by us today are giving us excessive weight and health problems, the diet consumed by our ancestors mainly contained lean meats, vegetables, fruits nuts, seeds and very limited amounts of grains, along with a very active and simple lifestyle that helped them to maintain excellent health and optimal weight, while eating only two times a day.

Paleolithic era is the pre-historic time also known as the Stone Age, as it was characterized by use of many tools made from stones .This era extended from about 200,000 years to 10,000 years BC. Our caveman ancestors had biologically adjusted greatly to whole foods: plants, meat, seafood—all of these filled with nutrients, which our bodies are programmed to thrive on.

The people back then were mainly hunters and gatherers,

they did not cultivate crops like wheat to make bread nor had the luxury of going to the super market to pick-up a microwave dinner. But in spite of their limited choices and methods to cook them, human in that era not only survived but also thrived on this diet.

Later after 10,000 BC came the "Neolithic" era or new Stone Age which brought with it the farming or Agriculture. Compared to more than 200,000 years of Paleolithic ages, the agriculture era has existed only a fraction of the time in history which is quiet not enough time for the humans to evolve completely to eating grains like wheat and sugars. The farming was later followed by the industrialization of food. This industrialization of food resulted in foods with high starch and sugar content, chemically processed vegetable and seed oils, and other "processed" foods. Therefore it was not a coincidence that many modern diseases of humankind including, cardiovascular disease, autoimmune disorders, type 2 diabetes, and widespread obesity—emerged and spread globally at the same time as industrialized food.

Not only what we eat was influenced but industrialization also affected when we eat. The cultivation of grains led to cereals and all related products and thus the over whelming support for breakfast later followed by the promotion of eating several small meals in a day. Hence, most of us eat over and over again without our body needing it or giving it the chance to burn the stored fat reserves, which has really played a dominant role in the soaring over weight and obesity problems all around.

**Autophagy; a Nobel Prize Winning process**

In 2016, the Noble Prize in Physiology or Medicine was conferred on Yoshinori Ohsumi for his research in the autophagy mechanisms. The word *autophagy* takes it root from the Greek words *auto-*, meaning "self", and *phagein*, meaning "to eat". Thus, autophagy means "self-eating". On the surface it sounds like an awful thing, our own body cells are doing to us, not after you understand what this process actually signifies.

The process of autophagy entails our cells recycling the unwanted parts like damaged proteins and attacking microorganisms and toxic compounds and removing them. This means that autophagy helps in slowing the aging process, and preventing diseases like cancer. There are factors that trigger this autophagy process and these include fasting, protein restriction, and carbohydrate restriction. It shows why intermittent fasting is an eating pattern that improves your health in so many ways.

Even before the awarding of Noble prize to Yoshinori Ohsumi, there were other researchers working on the benefits of autophagy for quite some time. In an article published in journal Cell Metabolism in 2007, authors showed that autophagy is essential for making muscle mass. The research team showed that how deactivating the autophagy gene resulted in the significant loss of muscle mass and strength.

This transpired as autophagy is essential for clearing-out of damaged proteins and mitochondria (energy store houses) in muscle cells. In absence of autophagy the damaged proteins and mitochondria will remain in the body and cause death of muscle cells, leading to a loss in muscle and strength. Nowadays, decluttering has become a buzz word, and people believe that decluttering their homes of unwanted things bring peace and harmony in their life, you can relate it to autophagy. This process declutters your body of long lying damaged cells so that you can have a renewed, energetic body system. It happens contrary to the belief that some nutrients will repair the damage, it actually involves changing your pattern of eating.

## Chapter Four

# Intermittent Fasting Methods

There are many different methods of doing intermittent fasting, however all of them are based on the basic principle that you split your day or week in to fasting and eating periods. You does not eat at all or only eat very little during fasting period, while you can eat anything during eating period but the key is to eat sensibly (we will talk about it in detail in later sections).

Some of the most popular methods of intermittent fasting are:

## THE 16/8 METHOD

This method is also known as daily intermittent fasting or the Lean gains protocol. This method involves a daily eating period of 8 hours and then you follow the fast for 16 hours.

This method essentially involves skipping one meal only- usually breakfast for most people, and is the most widely used method used for intermittent fasting.

## WEEKLY INTERMITTENT FASTING METHOD

It is also known as Eat-Stop-Eat method. This involves fasting for 24 hours, once or twice a week, for example by not eating from lunch one day until lunch the next day. Some people also do this method only once monthly. This timetable has the benefit of permitting you to eat every day of the week while still earning the benefits of fasting for 24 hours. You are not likely to lose any weight by this method because you are only cutting out two meals every week, thus this method might not be very productive for people trying to lose weight but people who want to retain the present weight while gaining some health benefits from intermittent fasting  might be good candidates for this method.

Perhaps the greatest advantage of doing a 24–hour fast is to get over the psychological fear of fasting. For people who have never fasted before, successfully completing  one 24 –hour fats helps them realize that not eating for one day won't kill them and they become ready to incorporate the intermittent fasting in their life style.  There are many options where you can incorporate 24- hour fast in your schedule like on a long day of traveling or on a day after a big celebration feast.

# THE 5:2 DIET

This method entails that you eat normally for 5 days and then restrict calories to only 500-600 for two non-consecutive days. Simply put you choose any two days in a week when you eat very less (recommended is 500 calories per day for women and to 600 calories/ day for men), while on remaining 5 days you eat as normal.

You can pick any two days of the week you like, but there has to be at least one non-fasting day in between them.

For instance you can eat normally on Sunday then fast on Monday with restricted calories, then eat normally for Tuesday and Wednesday and again fast on Thursday with 2-3 very small meals, , again you can eat normally for Saturday and Sunday.

The problem with this diet pattern is not with the method itself but with how you define and follow your "normal eating". My best guess is that who is over-weight and trying to find a way to lose some pounds is usually not in a habit of eating very healthy. Thus if normal eating means binge eating, processed foods, sweets and junk food, then in all probabilities you won't lose any weight with this method rather you will even gain some weight(*shudders*)

## ALTERNATE DAY INTERMITTENT FASTING

This method incorporates longer fasting periods on alternate days throughout the week.

For example, if you eat dinner on Sunday night and then not eat again until Monday night, when you will eat dinner. On

Tuesday, however, you would eat all day and then start the 24–hour fasting cycle again after dinner on Tuesday evening. This method lets you have long fasting durations on a consistent basis while you also get to eat at least one meal on each day of the week.

This type of eating is usually used in research studies about intermittent fasting. In reality following this pattern is less popular than other methods because not eating for almost 24 hours on alternate days needs lot of determination and people who are battling with weight issues as well as sugar addiction(yes, its true sugar addiction is a reality), comfort eating etc. might not have the resolve to fast for 24 hours. On the other hand, people who are happy with their weight and want to do fasting for health benefits would find it increasingly difficult to teach themselves to eat consistently more on the non-fasting days. It would require lot of planning, a lot of cooking and consistent eating. Thus, they end up eating the same amount of meals in their eating days although they are fasting for 24 hours on alternate days.

Therefore, the 16/8 method is the most feasible method both for people trying to lose weight and also who want to benefit from intermittent fasting while maintaining their present weight.

Let's talk about this method in more detail.

## WHAT IS THE 16/8 METHOD?

As we stated earlier, this method uses a period of 16- hour fast followed by 8-hours window of eating. This method is also famous by the name of daily intermittent fasting method or lean gains method. This name was popularized by Martin Berkhan, who propagated it through the website; Leangains.com.

The method is the considered to be less constrictive, most easy, convenient and sustainable intermittent fasting routine when compared to other methods.

It involves consumption of food and calorie-containing drinks for a period of 8-hours followed by 16 hours window of food abstinence.

You can repeat this cycle as frequently as you like- from every day to once or twice every week, it depends on your personal preference and your health/weight goals. Moreover, the method does not prescribe any specific eating or fasting hours. You can start your eating hours from any time you like, for example you may start at 8am and stop at 4pm. Or you can start at 2pm and stop at 10pm.

Most of the people following this method tend to find that eating between 1:00 PM to 8:00 PM works well for them because they feel that they only miss or delay breakfast and they can have lunch and dinner with their family and friends. Breakfast is usually a mealtime that people eat on their own, so skipping it isn't a big deal. Secondly, people who don't feel like eating early in the morning or don't have time for preparing breakfast because of their daily schedule really find it exciting to follow this schedule.

You can keep record of your eating and fasting hours in a table like the following:

## 16/8 Intermittent fasting method

| Time | Sunday | Monday | Tuesday | Wednesday |
|------|--------|--------|---------|-----------|
| 11:00 PM till 6:00 AM | Fasting and sleeping | Fasting and sleeping | Fasting and sleeping | Fasting and sleeping |
| 6:00 AM To Noon | Fasting | Fasting | Fasting | Fasting |
| Noon Till 8:00 PM | Eating | Eating | Eating | Eating |
| 8:00 PM till 11:00 PM | Fasting | Fasting | Fasting | Fasting |

| 16/8 Intermittent fasting method | | | |
|---|---|---|---|
| **Time** | **Thursday** | **Friday** | **Saturday** |
| **11:00 PM till 6:00 AM** | Fasting and sleeping | Fasting and sleeping | Fasting and sleeping |
| **6:00 AM To Noon** | Fasting | Fasting | Fasting |
| **Noon Till 8:00 PM** | Eating | Eating | Eating |
| **8:00 PM till 11:00 PM** | Fasting | Fasting | Fasting |

From the above table you can realize that if you eat in the window between 12 noon to 8:00 PM and in a habit of sleeping for 7 hours (ideally you should), then out of your fasting period you are sleeping for 7 hours and your actual fasting hours only remain to be 9 hours. Isn't it great? That's why this method is deemed as most doable and sustainable over a longer period of time, rather you can adopt as your life style. Since 16/8 fasting is done every day, getting into the habit of eating and fasting in this schedule becomes quite easy. Actually, right now you are accustomed to eating around the same time every day without giving it much conscious thought. With intermittent fasting it's almost the same thing, you just learn not to eat in a certain period of time, and it is remarkably easy once you are determined and can maintain consistency for few weeks. Once you are well- adapted to this routine over a period of time, wavering from it sometime won't hurt much until you come back to track soon. One intermittent fasting follower once wrote:

*"This is probably a good time to mention that while I have practiced intermittent fasting consistently for the last year, I'm not fanatical about my diet. I work on building healthy habits that guide my behavior 90% of the time, so that I can do whatever I feel like during the other 10%. If I come over to your house to watch the football game and we order pizza at 11pm, guess what? I don't care that it's outside my feeding period, I'm eating it".*

For the last decade or so, a lot of research effort is geared towards studying effects of intermittent fasting. The most studied form of time-restricted fasting is Ramadan fasting, which involves approximately 1 month of complete fasting (both food and fluid) from sunrise to sunset. Results show that there is significant weight loss which includes both reduction in fat mass as well as lean mass.

Another study compared eating one meal per day to three meals per day for 8 weeks and found that eating one meal was associated with fat loss and lean mass gain, while no significant improvements were detected in the 3-meal group.

# Chapter Five

# Who should be careful or avoid intermittent fasting?

I t goes without saying that intermittent fasting can do wonders for people wishing to lose weight or follow a healthy lifestyle, but at the same time it's not something that everybody needs to do. No doubt that it's one of the lifestyle patterns that can give you healthy benefits but we cannot undermine the importance of other factors that is your food choices, sleep and exercise. Secondly, it is not "one size fit all" solution, despite humongous benefits, there are people who should be careful about intermittent fasting or avoid it at all.

Intermittent fasting is great for some people, but not all. The only way to find out which group you belong to is to try it out. If you feel good and think that you can sustain intermittent fasting then it can prove to be a very powerful tool to lose weight and improve your health. But if you feel the opposite then you will have to look for a nutrition strategy to your liking and to which you can adhere.

The main side effect that most of the people experience on intermittent fasting is hunger. `Along with it you may feel some weakness and your brain might not seem to perform very well. All these side effects are mostly temporary as your body is trying to adjust to your new eating schedule.

There are groups of people who need to be careful or better avoid intermittent fasting including:

- People who are underweight

One potential disadvantage of 16/8 method is that when you typically cut out a meal or two out of your day, it gets difficult to get the same number of calories in during the week. Because not everyone can teach himself to eat bigger meals on a consistent basis. So, this eating pattern results in most of the people losing weight, which is a good thing for people who aim to lose weight. But for people who are already underweight, this can bring some health issues, and they better avoid this schedule.

- People with a history of eating disorders

People who have any eating disorder should consult with their doctor before trying to indulge in fasting. It is very important to understand that sometimes people with eating disorders may refrain from eating under the guise of intermittent fasting. These people tend to eat less or unhealthy even during the eating time period and eventually lose more weight and can develop many health complications.

- People with diabetes

Even though intermittent fasting may help in losing weight, which may help in    better control of diabetes, but it's important for diabetics to consult their health care team before embarking on journey of intermittent fasting. Together with the health team, they can decide what's most sustainable and safe for them as an individual. Especially for those with poor control of diabetes, full-blown intermittent fasting might not be a good idea due to the risk of blood sugar swings. In its place, you can reduce your portion sizes, increase your physical activity between meals, and make healthy food choices as an alternate approach.

Initially health care experts were vehemently against use of intermittent fasting    by people with diabetes. However, animal studies showed that intermittent fasting actually improved the function of pancreas in mice.

In an observational study, published in April 2017 in the World Journal of Diabetes, it was shown that  short-term daily intermittent fasting  may help to improve fasting and  post-meal glucose levels as well as control  weight and improve insulin sensitivity in people with type 2 diabetes. Although, it was a small study with only 10 participants and not a randomized controlled trial — the golden standard for research — the findings hold promise of intermittent fasting for diabetes patients. But more extensive research needs to be done to see if intermittent is truly safe for the larger group of people with type 2 diabetes.

*People with other medical conditions like low blood pressure and thyroid diseases (hyperthyroidism) and those on medications should also consult with their physician before starting intermittent fasting.*

## WOMEN AND INTERMITTENT FASTING

In research literature, there is some evidence that intermittent fasting may not be as beneficial for women as it is for men. For instance, in one study that compared glucose and insulin responses to a standard meal during intermittent fasting in both men and women. The results showed that insulin sensitivity improved in men, but blood sugar control worsened in women.

Although not many human studies are available in this regard but animal studies have found that intermittent fasting can make female rats masculinized, emaciated, and infertile and they miss their periods.

There are many anecdotal reports of women whose monthly periods stopped when they started doing intermittent fasting and they became normal after they went back to their previous eating pattern.

Because of these issues, it is advisable for women to adopt intermittent fasting with caution. Women should start slowly with smaller periods of fasting and advance in small increments. They should watch out for warning signs like amenorrhea (missing periods) and stop immediately if it happens.

Moreover, pregnant women and women who have fertility issues and those trying to become pregnant and lactating mothers are also groups that should avoid doing intermittent fasting

Having said all, it's still very true intermittent fasting has an excellent safety profile. If you are healthy and well-nourished, there is nothing dangerous in not eating for few hours every day or every week.

# Chapter Six

# Intermittent fasting:
# Separating Facts from Myths

In this age of information and technology, it's easier to get know- how on any topic you desire (thanks to Google). But in this information tide, sometimes the scientific knowledge is undermined and hearsay and half-cooked knowledge gets spread. You need to learn the actual facts and know how to separate myths from facts.

Here I would talk to you about few things which are very prevalent about fasting, but are not actually true.

1. Fasting slows down your Metabolism

You might have heard that with fasting you go into starvation mode and thus the metabolism slows. The answer is; no it does not. On the contrary, research studies have shown that short term fasting actually improve your metabolism, it's only if you are not eating for three or more days that your metabolism gets suppressed to conserve energy.

What we call starvation mode is actually natural response of our body to     compensate for drastic reduction in calorie intake over prolonged period of time. More scientific name for the process is adaptive thermogenesis. This natural mechanism has kept the human race from becoming extinct as it went through times of natural disasters, wars and much more. On intermittent fasting, if you are losing lots of weight, your body will try and conserve energy by burning less calories, but it will not stop you from losing down, it will only slow down your further weight loss to some extent.

TIP: *If you feel that you have reached a plateau and not losing weight any further due to possible slower metabolic rate, it's advisable to give your fasting a rest of 2 weeks. Scientific studies have shown that 2 – week break from intermittent fasting gives a boost to the metabolism and you start losing weight again. You have to be vigilant about not over eating in this 2 week break period, eat consciously and sensibly so that you don't end up putting on any weight that you have initially gotten rid of.*

2. You lose muscle mass when fasting

When you don't' eat during fasting, the fat stores in the body break down for energy, however some muscle break down also takes place and this loss of muscle mass may decrease the metabolic rate.

However, this process takes place when you are well into your weight loss journey, most of the people experience it after they have lost first 5-10% of their weight, occurring after about 3-6 months of intermittent fasting.

The good thing about intermittent fasting is that it helps preserve the muscle mass. In conventional dieting methods or calorie-reduction methods, 25% of weight loss is from muscle mass, while 74% is from fat loss, in comparison with intermittent fasting only 10% of weight drop is from loss of muscle mass and 90% is from fat loss.

In one research study the timing of eating was changed for participants from eating three times daily to one large meal in the evening without changing the amount of calories they were consuming. At the end of the study period it was observed that these people had significant reduction in fat and more importantly considerable increase in muscle mass along with improvement in other health markers (blood sugar, blood lipids etc.). For these reasons intermittent fasting is very popular amongst body builders because they find it effective for keeping low fat percentage in body while maintaining high muscle mass.

Here are some tips for you to ensure that you maintain your muscle mass during intermittent fasting:

- Increase your protein intake: You should try and incorporate higher amounts of proteins in your diet to avoid loss of muscle mass and thus slowing down of metabolism. Your goal should be to eat around 50 grams of proteins on your fasting day and 100 gram when you are not fasting. Moreover, the proteins in your diet will help you to feel fuller for a longer period and protect you from being over –indulgent and consuming lots of calories in your eating window.

- Lifts weight to build muscles: Resistance training is deemed to be the best method for keeping your metabolic rate higher. Lifting weights as part of your regular exercise regimen during intermittent fasting will help you to preserve muscle mass and may also add muscle mass. . Researchers compared the effect of resistance training and cardio exercise in women on intermittent fasting and found that women who did resistance training were able to maintain their metabolic rate while it slowed down for the group of women doing cardio exercise.

3. Eating frequent meals help you lose weight

One of the eating trends that has been trumpeted in recent years is that eating frequent meals boosts up your metabolism. This is also known as 6 meals a day regimen. This method became popular and accepted by fitness instructors, wellness professionals and others. People blindly followed this method without any scientific evidence of its effectiveness. When researchers probed this issue through scientific studies, it revealed that meal frequency has no effect on weight loss, neither it increases metabolism nor reduces hunger. For instance, a study in 16 overweight men and women compared the effect of eating 3 or 6 meals per day on weight, fat loss, and appetite. The study found no difference between the groups eating 3 or 6 meals per day.

The main reason people embraced 6 meals routine is that they were made to believe that it stokes the metabolic rate, so your body burns more calories.

The actual fact is that our body does need some energy to

metabolize the food we consume this is called the thermic effect of food, or TEF. The TEF varies for different food groups being 20-30% of calories for protein, 5-10% for carbs and 0-3% for fat calories. On average, around 10 % of the total calorie intake is used for total thermal effect. Thus, eating does increase the metabolic rate, but it depends upon the total calories that you consume and not on the number of meals; for example, if you consume 3000 calories per day either as 6 meals of 500 calories each or 3 meals of 1000 calories, the total calories used for TEF would be 300(10% of 3000) in both scenarios.

There has been numerous human studies that showed that increasing or decreasing meal frequency does not affect the total calories that are burned.

4. Intermittent Fasting is harmful for Health

Some people believe that fasting may have bad influence on the health, this idea is based on presumptions and is farthest from truth. Fasting in one form or the other has been in practice in humans and can be traced into pre-historic times. The ancient philosophers and experts wrote about its benefits and in modern times, there are plentiful animal and human studies that have shown that intermittent fasting actually has numerous health benefits.

We have already discussed these health benefits in earlier section of this book; just to give you a recap; Intermittent fasting  alters the gene expression in a way that you may live longer and have better protection from diseases. It can help to improve your metabolic health with better insulin sensitivity, reduction in oxidative stress and free radicals and decrease in chronic inflammation. All of these factors pitch in to decreases your risk of major health issue most importantly heart diseases.

Intermittent fasting also has beneficial effects for mental health as it boosts the brain hormone known as brain-derived neurotrophic factor (BDNF), this brain hormone protects against depression and other brain related issues.

5. Intermittent Fasting results in over eating afterwards

Many opponents of intermittent fasting try to propagate the impression that intermittent fasting actually makes you gain weight because you tend to over eat during the eating period. This might be partly true, people try to compensate for the calories they lost during the fasting period, by eating more during the eating period.

However, in most cases this compensatory eating usually is not even enough for making up for the calorie deficit. In a research study, it was shown that persons who fasted for one entire day, ate only 500 extra calories the next day. It means that in an average 2500 calories diet, they did not eat one day and ate 500 extra calories the next day but in total they were still about 2000 calories deficient for 2 days.

Intermittent fasting decreases overall diet consumption whereas improving metabolism at the same time. Many factors responsible for weight gain are also tackled during the fast such as; decrease in insulin levels, rise of norepinephrine level and increase up to 5 times in human growth hormone levels. All these factors make you lose weight while practicing intermittent fasting, this is verified by scientific evidence, a review study in 2014, showed that fasting for 3-24 weeks caused a loss of 3-8% in body weight and 4-7 % decrease in tummy fat.

Having said that, it's always advisable to watch what you eat during your eating window so as to reap maximum benefits out of intermittent fasting. I am sure our meal plans and recipes in the later part of this book would help you greatly to choose your food items.

6. Our body can process only a limited amount of protein in each meal

There are people who claim that our body can use only limited amount of proteins per meal (around 30 gms). Thus, we should eat every 2-3 hours in order to make sure that we have enough proteins for muscle gains. I don't know from where people get this idea, but it's definitely not based on scientific facts.

The studies done in this regard did not establish any difference in muscle mass if you eat proteins more frequently or in one or two meals per day.

The researchers concluded that it is the optimal amount of protein consumed that is essential for muscle building and it is not affected by the frequency of meals. So there is no need to eat proteins every 2-3 hours.

7. Frequent snacking is Good For Health

People who believe and publicize frequent eating are big supporters of more snacking throughout the day, they have also coined another term for it that is food grazing. You will find many articles on internet talking about grazing food and how it's good for health.

This concept is faulty from its foundation because human

body is not naturally programmed to be in fed state or simply grazing whole day. During evolution, passing through many eras like Stone-age, our ancestors went through many times of going without eating or very scarce eating.

The human race survived all these periods unscathed because short-term fasting starts a cell repair process in our body called autophagy; in this process body when missing the continuous flow of calories over a short period uses the old and non-functional stores of proteins as energy source.

In addition, fasting from time to time has many other health benefits as well. While on the other hand very frequent eating and snacking has been found to have negative health effects and also increase risk of various diseases. For instance in a research study it was found that frequent snacking lead to more deposition of fat in liver, a condition known as fatty liver. There are other studies suggesting that people who eat more frequently have increased risk of developing colorectal cancer.

There is also a danger of eventually consuming much more calories than you should while eating frequently. If you are having a snack too often, you try to keep the caloric value of each snack very low like 200-300 calories, but none of these will have any satiety value and you will end up eating more by the end of the day. It has been observed that people who are into snacking frequently also finish their day with a large dinner.

Eating too frequently does not give your body enough time to digest and process what you have eaten earlier. This affects protein synthesis- your ability to repair and build muscles- because you need the amino acids levels -the building blocks of proteins- to rise and then fall, which is not possible in a continuous fed state.

8. Brain function requires continuous Supply of Glucose

Some individuals are under the impression that if we don't' continuously provide glucose to our brain-in form of carbs, it will stop working. This perception has its roots in the belief that human brain can only use glucose (sugar present in blood) as energy source. However, the missing part in this argument is that this glucose does not always have to come from dietary sources, our body can easily produce needed glucose through a process called gluconeogenesis. Even before starting this process, our body can have sustained glucose levels for brain functioning by using glycogen (stored glucose in the liver).

Moreover, during fasting or on a very low–carb diet, the body can burn fat stores to produce ketone bodies. These ketone bodies can also be used as a fuel for brain functioning reducing the need for glucose. Therefore, the body can well maintain its brain function during fasting, using ketone bodies and glucose produced from proteins and fats.

9. Intermittent fasting increases Hunger

Some people believe that intermittent fasting increases hunger and frequent eating and snacking helps control cravings and excessive hunger.

Several studies have looked in to it and there are mixed views. Some studies agree with the idea that frequent snacking control hunger, while others suggest that there is no effect on hunger, conversely others showed that frequent eating actually increases hunger.

Along with frequency the macronutrients in our diet also matter a lot, when it comes to hunger. A study examined high protein meals eaten in 3 meals and 6 meals per day routine. Results revealed that 3 meals were better in controlling hunger.

10. Skipping Breakfast causes weight gain

For many years now, it has been drummed by all and sundry that breakfast is the most important meal of the day and the people skipping breakfast are the one becoming obese, unhealthy and have food cravings the whole day.

People quote many studies that found significant link between skipping breakfast and weight gain, but I would accept these results with a pinch of salt. Firstly, because these studies were observational meaning they were not good enough to establish a cause-effect relationship. Secondly, most of the people who skip breakfast usually have an overall unhealthy attitude towards eating. So, it's not skipping breakfast but what they eat the entire day that makes then obese/ overweight. This point was recently settled by a randomized controlled trial (the gold standard of research studies). The trial compared 283 overweight and obese adults in two groups; one eating breakfast and other skipping breakfast. After a follow-up of 4 months it was found that both groups have no difference in weight. Thus it' not something magical about the time, the benefits could be from what we eat in the breakfast. In 16/8 fasting method, you don't even need to skip breakfast, you need to only delay breakfast to 12:00 PM or another time according to your schedule. So if you are in habit of consuming very healthy breakfast, you can continue doing so with 16/8 intermittent fasting method, with just little tweak in the timings of your eating.

11. You can't exercise while fasting

We say that intermittent fasting is not a dieting method, it's a life style and no lifestyle could be healthy without inclusion of physical activity and exercise. It's very important that you maintain a good exercise routine during intermittent fasting (rather at all times)

Some time back people had hesitations in working out during fasting but with recent research it is evident that working out in a fasted state actually provide some additional benefits like burning more fat and building muscles.

It might be difficult in the start but soon you will adjust and find a balance. We will be telling you the tips and tricks of how to incorporate exercise in your intermittent fasting schedule in later part of the book.

.

# Chapter Seven

# Intermittent fasting and Keto diet

For the last few years there has been a lot of hype surrounding ketogenic or popularly known as keto diet, especially since many coveted names like Lebron James swearing about its effectiveness.

Intermittent fasting and ketogenic diet have a historical connection. In 1921, researcher Woodyatt showed that ketones appear in a normal person after a certain duration of fasting and also the same compounds appear in persons using a diet containing high proportion of fats and very low proportion of carbohydrates. At the same time, another researcher Dr Wilder in Mayo Clinic also suggested that the benefits of fasting can be obtained if ketosis can be achieved by use of high fat, low carb diet. Since then there are many diet experts who advocate the coupling of ketogenic diet and intermittent fasting so as to have better outcomes. Before discussing what these benefits are, let's look into what this ketogenic diet is.

# WHAT IS KETOGENIC DIET?

The ketogenic diet is a low carb, moderate protein and high fat diet that take its origin from two words; keto representing ketones and genic meaning producing. Ketones are the molecules formed by the liver in response to an absence of glucose (sugar), the body then burns these ketones as fuel for its energy requirements.

The ketogenic diet is based on the principle that by depleting the body of carbohydrates, which are its primary source of energy, you can force the body to burn fat for fuel, thereby maximizing weight loss. When we consume foods that contain carbohydrates, the body converts those carbohydrates into glucose, or blood sugar, which it then uses for energy.

Typically when we eat diet high in carbs, our digestive system breaks down these carbohydrates—into glucose, which is the simplest form of sugar that enters the bloodstream. In response to raised blood sugar levels, a hormone called Insulin is secreted by Pancreas, to drive the extra sugar into cells and use it for energy.

As glucose is the simplest and easiest molecule for our body to convert and use as energy, it is the preferred form of energy source. By choosing glucose as the energy source, the fats are usually not needed and remain stored.

By decreasing the carbohydrate intake, the body can be induced into a state known as ketosis. Ketosis is actually a natural compensatory mechanism of the human body to survive when food intake is low. During this phase, the fats in the liver are broken down to produce ketones. By ensuring a properly maintained keto diet, you can enter the same metabolic state; not by decreasing the calories but by restricting the carbohydrates intake. When body start using ketones as primary energy source, it offers many health benefits including decreased triglyceride levels, increased high density lipoproteins ( good cholesterol), good control of blood glucose and insulin and the visceral fat( layer of fat around the body organs) literally melts away.

It is important to remember that this is Nutritional ketosis and must not be confused with ketoacidosis. Ketoacidosis is a dangerous complication of type 1 and type 2 diabetes in which there is very high levels of blood sugar and ketones as a result of insufficient insulin levels to bring the circulating glucose into the cell.

In a person with normal pancreas, very low intake of carbohydrate can't induce ketoacidosis because even a very minimal insulin amount is enough to keep the ketones level in a safe range.

Having said that, there are certain high risk groups of people that should not try experimenting with nutritional ketosis unless they are under professional supervision; these include' type 1 diabetic patients, pregnant women and people with kidney disorders.

## POTENTIAL BENEFITS OF PRACTICING KETO DIET AND INTERMITTENT FASTING TOGETHER

If you plan to do the ketogenic diet whereas doing

intermittent abstinence additionally, it might provide the subsequent advantages:

## May swish Your Path to ketosis

Our bodies are programmed in a way that they can use various sources of energy including fatty acids, glucose, ketones, and alcohol. The choice of fuel to burn for energy depend upon availability; whatever is more in quantity will be burned more.

Following a low-carb, high-fat, moderate protein ketogenic diet places you into a state of ketosis. However, one of the main aims of the ketogenic eating style is to become keto-adapted. It means that your body is tailored to function with very less glucose.

After following keto diet for few days, your body enters into ketosis using fat for energy production, but initially the amount is low because of lack of fat-converting enzymes in your body. The enzymes involved in fat breakdown are completely different from the enzymes used in glucose break down. Typically, body is more accustomed to using glucose converting enzymes and needs sometime to adapt to cater for the increased demand of fat converting enzymes. This is also one of the reasons of people feeling of tiredness at the start of the ketogenic diet. When the enzyme built up has reached the required level, your cells change the way they acquire energy and you achieve keto adaptation. The duration of keto-adaptation process varies between individuals and may take from few weeks to few months. In keto-adaptation, your body's preferred fuel is fatty acids and its substrates (ketone bodies), and the beneficial effects reveal in form of more balanced hormone levels, glycogen stores in liver and muscles are depleted and there is less water retention. The energy levels also return back to normal again.

Intermittent fasting might facilitate your body reach ketosis faster than the keto diet alone. That's because during fasting your body, maintains its energy balance by shifting its fuel supply from carbs to fats — the precise premise of the keto diet During intermittent fasting , the hormonal levels are balanced and fat stores deplete leading your body to naturally begin burning fat for fuel.

### You lose more fat

Intermittent fasting and keto diet both help in losing fat, combining these two not merely adds there effect but multiplies it. The synergistic effect really punches the fat store very hard. Intermittent fasting boosts up your metabolism to produce heat (thermogenesis) that burns fat stores, similarly, fat stores are consumed during keto diet as fuel for energy.

Moreover, intermittent fasting helps to preserve muscle mass during weight loss and increase energy levels which helps keto dieters to increase athletic performance and remove body fat.

### Your hunger is suppressed

When you consume keto diet while on intermittent fasting, you can avoid one problem that is often experienced during fasting-Hunger. Research shows that a ketogenic diet suppresses hunger. The ketones produced during keto diet control the production of a hormone known as Ghrelin that boosts appetite. On keto diet, the ghrelin keeps at a lower level, even when you have not eaten for a long period. Thus, the keto food that you have devoured in dinner will help you get through the 16 hours fasting period without the hunger pangs.

### Your food cravings are controlled

Foods rich in carbohydrates like starch and sugar increase your hunger and food cravings and evading them keeps it at an adequate level. When you eat simple carbohydrates like sugar, it causes the blood sugar to rise. In response pancreas secretes Insulin, to drive the extra sugar into cells. The insulin receptors in cells containing glucose have to be clear for the proper action of the hormone. If this process is faulty, insulin resistance develops and as glucose is not able to enter cells, it stays in the blood. Now as the cells are not getting the fuel and energy for their function, they keep signaling to the brain for more release of insulin, resulting in sugar cravings. These persistent increased blood glucose levels also contribute in developing type 2 diabetes On the other hand foods rich in fats does not raise your blood sugar levels. The effect is profound and has been validated through a research study that it resulted in type- 2 diabetics getting off their medications. Consuming high fats and low carb diet will help you to ease in to intermittent fasting avoiding the hurdles of the cravings, fatigue, and mood swings that might make your fasting journey difficult.

# Chapter Eight

# Intermittent fasting and workouts

Earlier in this book, I have touched upon how exercising is important with intermittent fasting. Researchers have done several studies on exercises while fating such as on Muslim athletes in Ramadan and have found that fasting and workouts together can be done without any worry and rather have many benefits including:

- Better metabolic adjustments- research studies have shown that if you are training in fasted state you will have better hormonal profile including low insulin, more growth hormone and epinephrine.

- Increased muscle mass – Scientific evidence indicates that gain in muscle mass is increased when you combine fasting and physical activity. You train in fasted state and then have adequate nutrition during the eating period.

- Better absorption of nutrients during eating period-research studies have shown that if you work out in the fasted period, your body responds well to the post-workout meals. The food nutrients are well absorbed and bring better results.

## IMPORTANCE OF EXERCISE

We know that human bodies are designed for physical work and one needs to be physically active to remain healthy. Physical activity has a major positive effect in decreasing insulin resistance and it makes your tissues more sensitive for insulin.

Any kind of physical activity can play a significant role to make your insulin work but evidence shows that combination of aerobic activities — such as brisk walking, swimming, and cycling with resistance training, or weight training, seems to have the greatest benefit. Aerobic activities help in burning calories (and glucose) in every session of the exercise, while resistance training builds muscle, at the expense of the fat, this helps in utilizing glucose during exercise. As we have already discussed earlier, intermittent fasting isn't merely about what you eat, it's also about how you live. Active lifestyle, adequate exercise, sleeping 7–8 hours a night, and managing your stress are also important steps you can take to lose fat and prevent metabolic problems.

In terms of exercise following points would help you tailor and follow a daily fitness program that suits your needs:

- Target 30 minutes of activity every day: Most important for you is to remain up and moving, if you can do exercise in a stretch of thirty minutes that is well and good but you can break your exercise in several small duration activities over the day that sum up to at least 30 minutes.

- Increase your overall activity: Increase your daily activity in general—such as walking or climbing stairs—rather than a specific type of exercise. However, beware that don't count on house chores or other daily activity as your only exercise. Usually, people overrate the amount of exercise they get and underrate the number of calories they eat.

- Invest in a pedometer: Your answer to the problem of not enough activity can lie with a pedometer. Research has shown that pedometers can act as motivation for physical activity, and people who used pedometers increased their activity by about 27%. Keep a goal of 10,000 steps a day (about five miles); even if the goal is not archived initially, it's important that you make daily small increments to achieve the goal.

- Find an exercise partner: Exercising and working out with a partner or a friend can keep you motivated as research points out. It acts as a stimulus for a conducive exercise environment and may keep you more compliant with your fitness regime.

- Join an exercise group if you feel that exercising on your own is something that you can't handle

- Be realistic and set achievable goals: Once you start following an active life style, be realistic in your expectations. The results of the exercise would start showing in a shorter span of time but don't expect overnight miracles.

- Target one behavior change at a time: As I said that intermittent fasting is a life style change but don't try and make all changes at one time. If you are starting intermittent fasting then work on it for at least 30 days before you start your exercise program, because starting all activities at the same time have the inborn danger of abandoning all of them at the same time as well.

Following is a guideline that would help you tailor your daily exercise activities:

1. For those who are completely INACTIVE or rarely do a physical activity, start by increasing daily activities that are part of our daily routines such as:

– Take the stairs instead of the elevator

– Limit TV watching time and hide the TV remote control

– Make extra trips around the house or yard

– Do some stretching while standing in waiting line and take stretching breaks after every half hour of working on a desk or in front of the computer

2. For those are active some of the time, but not regularly

Try and become consistent with your physical exercise

program and follow it 2-3 times per week. Find activities that you enjoy such as playing golf, bowling, and working in your yard. You may also plan activities in your day such as stretching exercises, yoga, weight training, push/pull-ups, crunches etc. Simply refer to some recommendations below (which you can easily search for their illustrations on sites like Youtube) and you'll be getting an incredible workout without shelling out megabucks for a gym or personal trainer:

For Warm-up (about 5-10 min):

- Calf Wall Stretch

- Hip External Rotation Stretch

- Adductor Wall Stretch

- Reach-Across Shoulder Stretch

- Overhead Reach

- Doorway Chest Stretch

- Quadriceps Stretch

For Cardio (about 10-15 min): Use whatever you have access to – if you have a home gym with cardio equipment like a treadmill or elliptical, use that. If you don't, try walking whenever you can or running in place or doing jumping jacks indoors.

For Mobility & Core work (about 10-15 min)

- Split-Stance Chest Mobility

- Reach, Roll, & Lift

- Squat Mobilization

- Mountain Climbers

- Shoulder Wall Slides

For strength (about 10 min)

- Inclined Kneeling Push-Ups

- Partial Bodyweight Squat

- Full Bodyweight Squat

- Wide-Hands Push-Up

For Cool-Down (about 10 min): For the last part of your workout, repeat the exact same flexibility exercises you did in the warm-up.

3. For those who are already active most of the time or at least four days each week

Mix and match from all the above mentioned activities to achieve goal of remaining active for 4-5 days per week. You can follow aerobic exercise like brisk walking, bicycling, swimming, skinning. Sports like soccer, hiking, basket-ball, tennis, martial arts, and dancing are good options for people already having somewhat active life style.

In spite of the activity level you can always opt for the following options to keep your self-moving:

-Walk the dog

-Deliberately take longer routes

-Park your car a block away from your office

-Reek leaves in your garden

-Walk to your grocery store

Your success in being consistent lies in changing your routine if you start to get bored. Explore new activities and above all of this try and enjoy your exercise and have fun.


## WORK-OUTS WITH 16/8 FASTING METHOD

Now, I will talk about some special considerations related to 16/8 fasting method and exercise.

- Exercise Timing

For making your work out more effective during 16/8 method, you need to consider your exercise timings. You can choose from any of the three times; before, during or after the eating window. The timing you choose will depend on your preference; working before the eating window in fasted state suits people who prefer to work out on empty stomach, while people who does not like working out empty stomach and also want to capitalize the post-workout nutrition can choose to exercise during eating period. People who want to exercise in fed state but can't find time during eating window can do it after the eating period finishes.

- Select workout based on your diet composition

Experts of nutrition and fitness say that it's important that you take into account your diet composition; the macros you are consuming before deciding your workout program. For instance it's better to do resistance or strength workout on the day you consume more carbohydrates, while go for cardio or HIIT (high-intensity interval training) on a lower carb day.

- Consume the right meals post- workout to build or maintain muscle

Usually it is advised to do your work out during your eating period because of the above reason. So that you can keep your nutrition at adequate level after the work out. For example if you lift heavy weights during your work out, you need to have high protein afterwards for building muscles. Experts' advice to have carbohydrates and approximately 20 grams of proteins half an hour after the work out.

Your choice of meal size, when you are breaking your fast will depend on whether you have just exercised or you plan to work out later in the day.

If you have just worked out- consume around 50-60% of your total calories for the day in this meal including macronutrients from all food groups including carbs, proteins and fats.

If you are planning to work out later- in this case consume 30-50% of your calories for the day in your first meal consisting of macronutrients from all food groups. This will save you handsome amount of calories to be consumed after your work out.

- Adequate water intake

It's important to remember that intermittent fasting does not mean to restrict water consumption, rather you should aim to increase your daily water intake. More so, when you are exercising. You need to keep hydrated during and after your workout.

- Maintain your electrolytes level

Electrolytes are essential minerals present in our blood, sweat and urine including, sodium, potassium, chloride, bicarbonate and calcium. You need to replenish these electrolytes after sweating such as during strenuous exercise. One good option is coconut water as it has high amount of these electrolytes without the excess calories and it also tastes good. Avoid drinking too much sports drinks as they are high in sugar content and may cause more harm than benefit.

- Listen to some Music

Listening to music when you exercise will not only while away your boredom- but it will also help to enhance the quality of your work out, by keeping you focused and increasing your stamina. The choice of music is very important as research has been done to assess the effects of music have showed that fast-paced music with a great beat to dance to tends to improve athletic performance while doing exercise. For example, participants increased their treadmill speed and distance travelled without feeling fatigued.

There is a plethora of workout playlists on sites like Spotify, Pandora, and YouTube – so if you don't feel like building your own, look for one that matches your favorite genre! Of course, your playlist may vary depending on your musical tastes, but here are 20 of our favorites to start you off!

1. "212" by Azealia Banks

2. "One More Time/Aerodynamic" by Daft Punk

3. "Dark Horse" by Katy Perry

4. "Shake Your Body (Down to the Ground)" by Michael Jackson

5. "Pump up the Jam" by Technotronic

6. "Harlem Shake" by Baauer

7. "Single Ladies (Put a Ring on It)" by Beyoncé

8. "Body Movin' (Fatboy Slim remix)" by the Beastie Boys

9. "Let's Go" by Calvin Harris & Ne-Yo

10. "Push It" by Salt-N-Pepa

11. "Turn Down for What" by DJ Snake & Lil Jon

12. "Times like These" by Foo Fighters

13. "Hard to Explain" by the Strokes

14. "Team" by Lorde

15. "Roadrunner" by the Modern Lovers

16. "Titanium" by David Guetta & Sia

17. "Everlong" by Foo Fighters

18. "I Love It" by Icona Pop & Charli XCX

19. "Pound the Alarm" by Nicki Minaj

## 20. "Don't You Worry Child" by Swedish House Mafia

- Listen to your body

The last but not the least piece of advice is that always listen to your body. Although working out and intermittent fasting may work for many people, but there would be some that may not feel comfortable doing any kind of workout during fasting.

If you start feeling dizzy or weak during workout, it might mean that are having low blood sugar and you may need to have a drink with carbohydrate and electrolytes immediately, later followed by a good nutritious meal. Always remember to consult with your physician before starting any nutrition or fitness program.

Having said all, let's not forget that what works for someone may or may not work for you. If you are feeling weak by exercising or your exercise is getting affected by fasting, you have to work around your fasting and working out regimen to see how you can tweak it to accommodate both. However if at some point your fasting can't cope with exercise, it's alright to stop it completely for some time before you are able to find a fine balance between the two.

# Chapter Nine

# Intermittent fasting and supplements

K eeping up with the tradition of every other thing about health, wellness and fitness, the use of supplements during intermittent fasting also has some varied views; some deem it an outright necessity, while others believe that you don't need any supplementation if you are consuming nutrient-dense diet even once in a day. We will give you a balanced view and facts along with suggestions for the supplements that can be beneficial during intermittent fasting.

Before deciding about the supplements you want to use there are few things you should consider;

1) It is true that you can get most of the micronutrients needed by your body from the food that you eat even only once or twice as in 16/8 IF method. But most of you would still need supplementation because you may be micronutrient deficient

because of earlier dietary habits, secondly it might be difficult to consume food that contains all the required vitamins and minerals on daily basis.

2) Only ingesting supplements is not enough, they need to be absorbed adequately for their beneficial effect. For example the vitamins that are fat soluble such as Vitamin D and Vitamin E need some fat containing food taken along with them for absorption ( thus can be consumed only during eating period) while other water soluble vitamins like vitamin B6 can be taken in fasting period.

3) If you happen to skip your supplements for a day or so, it will not put you at any high risk, as touted by some people. Rather there is a compensatory mechanism known a Hormetic effect which denotes that skipping micronutrients for a limited time will actually improve their absorption if you follow it up with high quality nutrition.

4) Remember not to over –load yourself with supplements; abundance of these supplements can be harmful as they may interfere in absorption of other nutrients from the food.

Some of the supplements that you can use during intermittent fasting are as follows;

- Mineral supplements containing electrolytes like sodium, potassium, magnesium are required because they are flushed from the body when you are burning fat stores for energy.

  You require at least 1500-2300 mg of sodium every day to avoid headaches and muscle cramps, this requirement increases to about 4000-7000 mgs, if you are physically active during fasting. The recommended daily requirement for potassium is about 1000-4700 mgs. Potassium deficiency can result in heart palpitations, increased blood pressure, muscle cramps and decreased energy. If you start feeling extremely tired during IF, low potassium could be the reason. For magnesium the daily required amount is about 300-450 mgs. Magnesium supplements in form of magnesium salt or flakes are available to be used to prevent and treat magnesium deficiency.

• Zinc and Calcium supplements can also be used in intermittent fasting. It is also important to remember that these minerals interact with each other and also compete for absorption. Thus if you are using magnesium then you should be cautious in using calcium because it inhibits the former's absorption. Similarly people with low hemoglobin (anemia) using iron supplements should not use zinc supplement concomitantly because it slows copper absorption which in turn slows iron absorption.

• B-Complex Vitamins including riboflavin, niacin, biotin, and thiamine are vital because they assist the body in absorbing nutrients. Vitamin B-complex supplementation is especially required for people already deficient in these and they also help in proper absorption of magnesium and potassium.

• Exogenous ketones; one of the most commonly used supplement from this group is Beta Hydroxybutyrate, or BHB. It is one of the three ketones produced naturally in the liver as your body enters ketosis. Using exogenous ketones is especially important for people combining intermittent fasting and ketogenic diet. At the cellular level, your body needs BHB, either from natural sources or from supplements, to burn the stored fats for energy production through the Krebs cycle. Using BHB supplement during IF will ensure that you have enough ketones in your blood stream to metabolize fat stores. BHB supplements are usually combined with potassium and magnesium to ensure adequate levels of required electrolytes.

• BCAA supplements; actual long name is Branched Chain Amino Acids, are very frequently used supplements in intermittent fasting method, particularly by those who wish to build muscle mass. BCAA supplements deliver the similar vital amino acids present in protein that permit your body to maintain and build muscle. Some people contend that BCAA supplements contain calories and can disrupt fast and put you out of fasting, however, these diet supplements do contain calories but they are only about six calories per gram and, thus do not pose any significant risk to your fast. Most of the individuals enjoy positive results with BCAA supplements and don't experience any negative effect to their fast.

In addition to all of the above, the best supplement you can use while fasting is H2O aka water. Yes water is one of the best things to be used during your fast. It will help your body tissue and internal organs including brain to function properly and sustain satisfactory levels of minerals and nutrients. Water also aids in eliminating toxins and wastes from your body properly. On the other hand dehydration can lead to tiredness, fatigue, irritability, confusion, muscle cramps, dizziness and cravings.

*It's important to discuss with your doctor before you choose the supplement you want to use while on intermittent fasting.*

# Chapter Ten

# Great Tips and Tricks for doing intermittent fasting

I f you have decided that intermittent fasting is the way of life you want to adopt, here are some key concepts and tips for easing your way into intermittent fasting and to maintain this life style successfully.

## 1. Make sure that intermittent fasting is the right approach for you

There is no doubt that intermittent fasting has considerable benefits for majority of people, but as we already said "it's not a one glove fit all 'type of solution. There are few groups' of people who might not be the right candidates for this method. You should take into account your lifestyle, nutritional and exercise experience before deciding to embark on the intermittent fasting journey.

## 2. Start slowly but steadily

Remember the famous saying " slow and steady- wins the race", when easing your way in to intermittent fasting, it's essential that you do slow in the start but remain firm and work your way up steadily. For example in 16/8 method; people already in routine of having widely-spaced meals can try 16 hours fasting from start, but if you are a person snacking frequently or having 5 -6 meals per day, it's better that you pick up small things like adjusting your usual meal time by an hour. See how it goes and then upgrade your method accordingly.

## 3. Give yourself some time

Intermittent fasting like any other lifestyle change will take some time before it starts showing results. Don't rush into it expecting some magic. You didn't put on all this weight by eating few meals, so don't expect to get it all off by skipping few meals. Keep your expectations realistic.

## 4. Start your fast post-dinner

This tip is especially effective for 16/8 method. Following this would mean that you spend a big portion of your fasting time asleep. For example, you can follow the following steps;

a) Have dinner at 8:00 PM

b) For next 2-3 hour do reading, watching TV, or any other evening activity

c) Sleep for 6- 9 hours

d) By the time you wake up you have already fasted about 2/3 rd. of the fasting period making 16 hours fast so much doable.

Keeping this schedule makes your lifestyle much simpler; you can manage hunger well and adhere to your eating: fasting schedule better.

## 5. Consume more fulfilling meals

In any diet, the foods that you eat are the decisive factor that can make or break your sticking to the diet. In this regard, intermittent fasting has a big edge above other type of diets. Imagine a usual fat loss diet; it would be eggs or cereal in breakfast followed by some bland grilled chicken or fish and veggies for lunch. After workout protein shake or water and a dinner similar to the lunch. If you are fortunate enough, you may scrounge some calories to throw in a handful or two of dry nuts. Such uninspiring food choices couple with the hunger and food cravings, are bound to falter you from your dieting track.

This is not the case with 16/8 intermittent fasting method. In a typical day, you can skip breakfast and have water, coffee or any other drink (no calories) that you want. At lunch time you can have grilled chicken but with much tastier accompaniments such as baked or mashed potatoes with veggies on the side with dressing. You can have a protein shake or water after work out. Dinner at around 8:00 PM could be homemade chicken casserole (recipe included in this book) or if you are invited to a party you can have anything you want even pizza but CAUTIOUSLY. If you are a big fan of breakfast food you can include omelets etc. in your lunch time or as snack's twice during the day. Another advantage of including satiating foods in your meals is that it helps you avoid hunger and cravings.

## 6.  Keep yourself busy

Most of us can relate to instances when we were so busy in office, at home or anywhere else that we totally forgot to eat. On the other hand boredom is your enemy in more than one ways. Beware of it before it curtails your progress and pulls you back from your track. Give it a thought; a slow day in office with nothing much to do and suddenly the snacks and coffee or a trip to cafeteria creeps in, or you are at home watching movie, which you don't like much, you get up and head to kitchen, open fridge and there goes your diet control.

But how boredom ends up in us eating?

The responsible for this is a chemical released from our brain; the dopamine. This is also known as the feel good chemical that makes us good sensation whenever we achieve a goal. Interestingly, eating also results in release of this chemical and thus the motivated behavior. Especially the foods which we call junk food including high salt, sugar, and fat containing foods are good at making us feel good. Researchers has done studies on this phenomenon and showed that persons who were bored consumed more calories as compared to those who weren't. It was further elucidated that this response was same in both normal weight and overweight individuals. So it's important that you keep yourself busy so as to avoid indulging in food unnecessarily.

## 7. Learn to blunt your hunger

It is expected that you will experience hunger pangs during fasting, especially at the start. Your success lies in handling these hunger pangs and the best way to blunt them is to drink water or other beverages with zero calories, it will help

71

you to feel full and keep hunger checked until it's time for you to break your fast. The drinks that you may consume include bubbly water, green tea, coffee, and tea (both without sugar and milk).

## 8. Eat in moderation when breaking fast

Although we touched upon it earlier, but need to say it again; remember not to treat fasting as an excuse to over eat. Thus when you are breaking fast you need to eat in moderation because you will achieve fat loss only when you maintain sufficient calorie deficit. When you skip breakfast and eating after a 16 hours fasts, it's understandable that it gives you more freedom to choose for your meal. BUT if you go overboard with your eating you are bound to lose the calorie deficit that you have worked hard to achieve. By achieving a good meal with adequate calories (without going overboard) will help you to stay on track and have sufficient calories to consume during rest of your eating window.

## 9. Maintain your Routine

Routine is defined as "a fixed way of doing things". Generally speaking, a person following a routine is thought to be "unexciting" or 'less innovative ", but when we talk about intermittent fasting, sticking to a routine is extremely important.

For developing a routing for intermittent fasting, you must find out what works for you and then stick to it so as to avoid confusion and second guessing.

It also helps you in avoiding decision fatigue. Decision fatigue simply means that after prolonged period of decision making, you eventually lose your ability to make decisions. You eventually get to point that you take the easier choice or wrong choice.

By following the same time for fasting and eating window, choosing some  meal plans for a week or 10 days and then repeating it all over again and similar measures helps reducing the decision that you have to make every day and removes the potential barrier to your success. It will mean that you don't have to make every day decision of what you'll eat, when you'll eat it, when you'll cook it etc.

## 10. Allow Yourself Time to Fine-tune in to intermittent fasting

It's only human to expect results right away, but it's not very realistic. How much we want to dodge the initial fumbling part of any thing and go straight to the pro phase or wish to pronounce "I know what I am doing". It's usually not the case in reality. Like everything else expect some teething problems when starting intermittent fasting.

You ought to grant your body some time to adjust to fasting, particularly if it is your first time. So if you are experiencing hunger pangs or slip up few times, it's only normal. It does not mean that you need to stop or it will not work for you. Conversely, it's an opportunity for you to learn, you need to do a self-evaluation to see what is the reason of these slip ups, and what steps you need to take to stop it from happening again. By doing so, you will be able to tackle the present problem as well as be better prepared for any future difficulties.

By going through this process you'll be better prepared for future difficulties that may arise in the future. But always remember don't give up and give yourself some time.

## 11. Be realistic

Some points need to be emphasized even at the cost of sounding like a broken record. Being realistic is one of them. The most common reason people yo-yo between different diets, fitness programs, wellness regimes, is that their expectations usually overrun what can be actually achieved in a certain amount of time.

Similar to all life style changes, intermittent fasting is neither a quick fix nor shortcut to reach your weight goals if nothing else is working for you. It's a dietary change that will work only if done correctly and will take some time to show visible results.

Remember that you didn't end up with this weight or body shape in a day, week or month, neither will you be able to regain your dream body shape that quickly. Be consistent and realistic.

## 12. Be ready for some deviations

It's evident that the whole world is not going on diet program with you. While you are following intermittent fasting you will still need to eat out with friends, attend parties and go on vacation. The advantage with intermittent fasting is that you can still keep on track while enjoying with your friends and family.

• By skipping breakfast , you already a create a calorie deficit of about 300- to 900 calories depending upon what you usually eat in breakfast

- If it's a birthday dinner in the evening; you can have your first meal as a protein filled lunch, skip the evening snack and you would be good to enjoy the party with enough calorie allowance in your account.

- While going on vacation; follow two meals policy, one in after noon and other in noon. Do lot of walk and enjoy your trip.

- As a general rule, apply 70:30 principle. Most of the food choices must be from nutritious foods with a mix of essential macronutrients and micro nutrients while a minority can be from foods you enjoy even if they are less in micronutrients and vitamins.

This will help you to tackle cravings, stick to intermittent fasting and keep your sanity.

# Chapter Eleven

# Meal plan and Recipes

I n the following section you will find meal plans and recipes to be used while doing 16/8 intermittent fasting method. Before giving the details of the meal plan and the recipes, there are few things, which are essential for you to know:

> As we discussed earlier, intermittent fating is more about when to eat than what to eat. But having said that, it's also true that IF is a life style change and when you are changing your life style, its better be a good change. Thus, the meal plans and the recipes included here are aimed to give you an idea about the ingredients, their quantity and cooking techniques that are desirable for maintaining a healthy diet. The meal plans have been divided into 7 day meal plans focusing different diet regimens and contain ideas each for breakfast, lunch, dinner and snacks. You can mix & match or may even

repeat the same recipe in same week or make the food in large batches to be used later during the week.

➤ A week meal plan for keto diet is also included as we know that when intermittent fasting and keto diet are combined, they bring much better and faster results. All of the recipes included in this week plan are strictly Keto. They are low-carb, grain-free, dairy-free (except for ghee), legume-free, soy-free (except for tamari sauce), and free of processed sugars and seed oils. We have kept the net carbs in these meals as less than 20g and calories range from 1400-2200., so that you can add coffee, other snacks or other desserts in your daily diet.

➤ You need to tailor the amount of food as well as the ingredients depending upon your likes (dislikes), allergies, lifestyle, exercise regimen etc. As a principle, drink lot of water and refrain from eating late night dinners.

➤ Most of the people following 16/8 intermittent fasting tend to skip breakfast and eat their first meal around 12 midday or later. But still it is not mandatory and people can have their eating window as they wish and can include breakfast time or have the breakfast as their first meal even if it is in the middle of the day. Plenty of breakfast ideas have been included in the meal plans for these people. However, mornings are usually busy and rushed for most of us that's why it's more advisable to try few recipes and choose the ones that you really like and stick to them. Leave your experimentation for lunch or dinner when you have more time at hand.

➤ All the recipes include the nutritional data including the total calories, total carbs, fiber, net carbs and protein. Please note that these figures are for one serving so even when you make large batches with double or more quantity, the nutritional value of each serving will remain the same.

➤ We have tried to provide you with a variety of recipes to make your intermittent fasting more varied and fun, but you can find many others on internet, just keep referring to the basic concepts; the carbs, fats, protein ratio, the food items with good nutritional value and you will soon be able to make your own personalized meal plans and recipes.

➤ We would also reiterate once again that aim of this book to help you live a fulfilled and happy life and that is more than just diet, your sleep, stress levels, social connections, exercise level all are very important and should be taken care of for benefiting from intermittent fasting to its fullest.

# MEAL PLAN: WEEK 1

| Day | Meal 1 | Snacks | Meal 2 | Total calories |
|---|---|---|---|---|
| 1 | Chicken vegetable salad | -Fruit of your choice -Protein bar | Spicy beef mix | 350+ 440 +95 + 550= 1435 |
| 2 | Grilled Fish with salsa | -I handful of mixed nuts -1 boiled egg | Burrito with Quinoa Salad | 450+200+ 155+ 600= 1405 |
| 3 | Vanilla Milkshake Smoothie | -Protein Bar -Fruit of your choice | Tuna filled Pitas | 328+440+ 100+575= 1443 |
| 4 | Garlic Chicken Drumsticks | -A handful of Almonds -Dark chocolate 1 piece | Pizza Stuffed Mushro oms | 1000+169+ 170+ 350= 1689 |
| 5 | Grilled Chicken burgers | -Yogurt with Vanilla, Cinnamon, Nutmeg, and Flax Seeds -Fruit of choice | Flank Steak | 600+200+ 100 +350=1250 |

| | | | | |
|---|---|---|---|---|
| 6 | Salmon With Apricot and Couscous | -I handful of mixed nuts<br><br>-1 boiled egg | Spinach and Tomato Pasta | 490+100+ 200+280= 1077 |
| 7 | Beef & Cabbage Stir-Fry With Peanut Sauce | -Fruit of your choice<br>-Protein bar | Cheesy Broccoli Soup | 450+440+ 100+ 250= 1240 |

# RECIPES

## Day 1

### 1. Meal 1: Chicken vegetable salad

Time required: for Preparation: 15 minutes| Cooking: 10 minutes

Skill level: Easy

You will need;

For the salad

- Chicken breast : 1

- Cooking oil: 2 tablespoons

- Edamame beans: 1 cup shelled, cooked according to package directions and cooled

- Bell peppers: 2 medium diced

- Carrots: 1 cup shredded

- Coleslaw mix: 4 cups tricolor

- Cilantro: 1/2 cup chopped

- Green onions: 3 thinly sliced

- Almonds: 1/4 cup toasted

- Sesame seeds: 1 tablespoon

For the dressing:

- Garlic: 1 teaspoon minced

- Soy sauce: 1/4 cup

- Rice vinegar: 2 tablespoons

- Honey: 1/2 tablespoons

- Pinch of ground ginger

- Salt and black pepper to taste

Method

1. Place a skillet on the stove and put 2 table spoons of oil. Finely chop the chicken breast and put in the heated oil and cook it thoroughly.

2. For making the dressing mix all ingredients including garlic, soy sauce, rice vinegar, honey, and ginger in a small bowl.

3. Take a large bowl and mix, edamame beans, bell peppers, carrots, and coleslaw with chicken. Toss well with a wooden spoon.

4. Now blend in the dressing into the salad so that salad is well coated with the dressing. Garnish with the cilantro, and mix again.

5. Sprinkle the green onions, toasted almonds, and sesame seeds on top, if desired.

6. You can eat immediately after preparation or keep it refrigerated for 1 hour for better taste.

| Nutrition Facts |
| --- |
| Total calories: 350 |
| Fat: 34 g |
| Total Carbs: 16 g |

## 2. Meal 2: Spicy Beef Mix

Time required: for Preparation: 15 minutes| Cooking: 30 minutes

Skill level: Medium

You will need;

- Cooking oil: 2 table spoon

- Onion: 1 finely chopped

- Green pepper: one diced

- Garlic, 2 cloves finely chopped

-  Jalapeños: 1 thinly sliced

- Mince beef: 1- pound

- Chili powder: 1 teaspoon or according to taste

- Tomatoes: 2 medium sized skin removed and finely diced

- Chicken stock: 2 table spoons

- Brown sugar: 1 tablespoon

- Apple cider vinegar:1 tablespoon

- Hot sauce: 1 tablespoon

- Salt: to taste

- Red kidney beans: 1 can drained

For garnishing (Optional)

- Cilantro: 1 tablespoon shredded

- Light sour cream: 1 tablespoon

- Mexican-blend cheese: 1 tablespoon shredded

Method

1. In a pan add 1 tablespoon of oil over medium to high heat in a large skillet, put mince beef and sauté it until meat is lightly browned. It will take approximately 5-7 minutes. Keep it aside

2. In a large skillet, heat cooking oil over high heat. Put in onions, peppers, jalapeños, and garlic. Lower the heat and cook vegetables for about five minutes, until they are tender and onions are translucent.

3. Now add mince beef — cook, stirring to break up lumps, for about 5 minutes. Add chili powder, and cook for minute.

4. Add tomatoes, chicken broth, brown sugar, vinegar, hot sauce, and salt. Reduce the heat and let the chili simmer over low heat for another 10 minutes. Don't forget to stir often.

5. Put in the beans; cook until heated through, for about 5 minutes.

6. Garnish with topping of your choice, and bon appétit!

| Nutrition Facts |
| --- |
| Total calories: 550 |
| Fat: 34 g |

| Total Carbs: 35 g |
| --- |
| **Protein: 54g** |

## Day 2

### 3. Meal 1: Grilled Fish with salsa

Time required: for Preparation: 10 minutes| Cooking: 20 minutes

Skill level: Medium

You will need;

- 1/4 cup water

- Firm white fish cutlets or fillets: 4 each weighing about 150gms each

- Olive oil cooking spray

- Asparagus: 1 bunch ends trimmed and cut into 3cm long pieces

- Lettuce: 1 bunch

- Cucumber: 1 medium sized coarsely chopped

- Lime wedges: to serve

For Salsa

- 2 large ripe tomatoes, sliced, deseeded, finely chopped

- 6 -8 olives, finely chopped

- 2 tablespoons finely shredded fresh basil

- 1 teaspoon olive oil

- 1 tablespoon fresh lime juice

Method

1. Preheat a chargrill or barbecue flat plate on medium.

2. Coat both sides of the fish with olive oil cooking spray. Season with pepper.

3. Cook on grill for 3-4 minutes on each side or until golden. Meanwhile, blanch the asparagus in a saucepan of boiling water for 1 minute, then place under running cold water.

4. Drain the asparagus and place with lettuce, snow peas and cucumber in a bowl and toss to combine.

5. To make the salsa, combine the tomato, olive, basil, oil and lime juice in a small bowl and season with salt and pepper.

6. Put fish in serving plates, top it with the salsa. Serve with lime wedges and the salad

| Nutrition Facts |
| --- |
| Total calories: 450 |
| Fat: 30 g |
| Total Carbs: 28 g |
| Protein: 56 g |

## 4. Meal 2: Burrito with Quinoa Salad

Time required: for Preparation: 15 minutes| Cooking: 40 minutes

Skill level: Advanced

You will need;

- Quinoa: 1 cup

- Water: 2 cups

- Olive oil: 1 tablespoon

- Onion: ½ chopped

- Red pepper, 1 diced

- Tempeh: 1 (8-oz.) package diced into bite-size pieces

- Salsa: 1 cup

- Lime juice: 1 tablespoons

- Cumin: 1 teaspoon

- Cayenne pepper: 1/4 teaspoon

- Black beans: d1 (15-oz.) can drained and rinsed

- Fresh or frozen corn: 1 cup

- Cherry tomatoes: :  1/2 cup halved

- Fresh cilantro: 2 tablespoons

- Salt and pepper, to taste

- Avocado, 1 diced

Method

1. Place a sauce pan with two cups water over high heat. Add the quinoa in water and cook in covered pot on high heat. As it starts to boil, reduce heat so it simmers and cook for another 20 minutes or until the water is absorbed and the quinoa is fluffy.

2. As the quinoa is cooking, prepare the tempeh. Place oil in a pan and heat it over medium heat. Add onions and cook for five minutes until they are soft. Now add the diced red pepper, tempeh, salsa, lime juice, cumin, cayenne pepper, and salt and pepper in the pan.

3. Keep cooking the tempeh mixture for another 15 minutes or so and keep stirring frequently.

4. When the quinoa and tempeh mixture are cooked thoroughly, transfer them into a glass bowl and blend together. Finally put the remaining ingredients; beans, corn, tomatoes, cilantro, and a little salt and pepper, and mix well.

5. You can enjoy it as such topped with few slices of avocado or can use as a filling for burritos.

| Nutrition Facts |
| --- |
| Total calories: 600 |
| Fat: 14 g |
| Total Carbs: 50 g |
| Protein: 18 g |

## Day 3

### 5. Meal 1: Vanilla Milkshake Smoothie

Time required: for Preparation: 10 minutes

Skill level: Easy

You will need;

- Soft tofu: 1/2 cup

- Vanilla soy milk: 1 cup

- Banana: 1 (frozen)

- Peanut butter: 1/2 tablespoon

Method

1. Put all ingredients in the blender and mix till you get a smooth mixture for about a minute.

2. Pour the smoothie in glass tumbler and. Enjoy!

| Nutrition Facts |
| --- |
| Total calories: 328 |
| Fat: 13 g |
| Total Carbs: 41 g |
| Protein: 18 g |

## 6. Meal 2: Tuna filled Pitas

Time required: for Preparation: 15 minutes

Skill level: Easy

You will need;

- Whole-wheat pitas: 2

- Tuna: 1 can, fish in water without salt

- Lemon juice : ½ teaspoon

- Olive oil: 2 teaspoons

- Red onion: ½ diced

- Red bell pepper: 1/2 cup diced

- Parsley: 2 tablespoons finely chopped

- Salt and pepper: to taste

Method

1. Open can of tuna, drain the water, and place tuna in a bowl.

2. Mix lemon juice and olive oil.

3. Add bell pepper, onion, and parsley. Also sprinkle salt and pepper according to taste.

4. Take the pita bread and stuff tuna filling inside it.

5. Fill in the second pita bread also and serve.

| Nutrition Facts |
|---|
| Total calories: 575 |
| Fat: 24 g |
| Total Carbs: 40 |
| Protein: 54 g |

# Day 4

## 7. Meal 1: Garlic chicken drumsticks

Time required: for Preparation: 30 minutes, cooking: 30 minutes

Skill level: Advanced

You will need;

- Chicken drumsticks: 10-12 with skin

- Olive oil: 2 table spoons

- Butter: 4 tablespoons

- Garlic: 3 cloves finely chopped

- Lemon zest: from 1 lemon

- Lemon juice: 1 table spoon

- Salt and pepper to taste

- Parsley: 2 table spoons for garnishing

Method

1. Season chicken drumsticks with generous amount of salt and pepper. Let the chicken sit at room temperature for at least half hour or more if time permits.

2. Before cooking, dry the drumsticks with paper towels.

3. Place a large heavy-bottomed, non-stick (preferable) skillet over medium heat. When skillet is heated add olive oil and half of the butter. When the butter is foaming, add drumsticks in a batch of 4 or 5 at a time and brown the

drumsticks on all sides. Keep the browned drumsticks in a large plate.

4. Now lower the heat and add all drumsticks back to the skillet. Cover the skillet with a lid and cook drumsticks on medium-low heat for 20-25 minutes. Flip the drumsticks and rearrange them every 5-7 minutes for even cooking on all sides.

5. Uncover the skillet and toss in the remaining ingredients including butter, garlic, lemon zest, and lemon juice. Gently mix to coat the drumsticks with the ingredients.

6. Remove the skillet off the heat and allow the chicken to rest for some time, it will also allow the flavors to infuse well. Garnish with parsley, and serve hot.

| Nutrition Facts |
| --- |
| Total calories: 1000 |
| Fat: 500 g |
| Total Carbs: 5 g |
| Protein: 120 g |

## 8. Meal 2: Pizza stuffed mushrooms

Time required: for Preparation: 10 minutes, cooking: 20 minutes

Skill level: medium

You will need;

- Portobello Mushroom Cups: 4

- Tomato Pasta Sauce: 2 tablespoons

- Grated Cheese: ½ cup

- Oregano: ½ teaspoon

- Salt and pepper: to taste

Method

1. Set your oven to preheat at 200C (400F). Take a baking tray and line it with either baking paper or foil.

2. Take off the stems from the mushroom cups and arrange them onto the prepared baking tray.

3. Place cheese, pasta sauce, oregano or any other topping of your choice on the mushrooms. Sprinkle salt and pepper.

4. Bake in the oven for 15-20 minutes or until the mushrooms are cooked to your liking.

5. Take out from the oven and enjoy.

| Nutrition Facts | |
|---|---|
| **Total calories: 350** | |
| **Fat: 25 g** | |
| **Total Carbs: 20 g** | |
| **Protein: 12 g** | |

## Day 5

### 9. Meal 1: Grilled Chicken burgers

Time required: for Preparation: 10 minutes, cooking: 10 minutes

Skill level: medium

You will need;

- Mince chicken: 200 gm.

- Fish sauce: 2 tablespoons

- Parsley : ½ bunch leaves only, chopped

- Sesame oil: 1 teaspoon

- Shallots: 1 thinly sliced

- Salt and pepper

- Burger buns: 2

- Yoghurt: 2 tablespoon

- Chipotle paste: 2 table spoon

- Sliced tomato and lettuce leaves to serve

- Sweet Potatoes: 2, cut in to fries

Method

1. Set your grill to preheat at the highest setting.

2. Put the chicken meat, fish sauce, coriander, sesame oil and spring onion into a large bowl. Season generously with salt

and pepper. Now dig your hands in the meat mixture and blend well. This way burgers will hold together better when grilled. Divide the meat into two equal portions and shape in to burger patties.

3. Transfer the patties on your grill pan or baking tray and grill the burgers for 5 minutes on each side or until they are completely cooked through. Slice into one of the patties to check if it is cooked through. The meat should be white all the way and no raw pink portions left.

4. In the meantime, slice the burgers bun into halves. Mix the chipotle paste and the yogurt and spread on the burger buns. Place the sweet potato fries in the microwave for 7 minutes at 900w, then leave to rest for 30 seconds. Heat the coconut oil in a frying pan over a high heat. Add the sweet potato fried and fry for about 3 minutes on each side or until they are nicely browned all over. Drain on paper towels, and then season with a good pinch of salt.

5. When your burger patties are cooked, remove from the grill and build your burger stacking it up with tomato and lettuce

| Nutrition Facts |
|---|
| Total calories: 600 |
| Fat: 48 g |
| Total Carbs: 20 g |
| Protein: 46 g |

### 10. Meal 2: Flank Steak

Time required: for Preparation: 15 minutes, cooking: 20 minutes

Skill level: medium

You will need

- Canola oil: 2 tablespoons

- Chicken broth: ½ cup concentrated

- Honey: ½ tablespoon

- Soy sauce: 1/2 cup low-sodium

- Green onions: 4, cut into thin, diagonal slices

- Fresh ginger: 1 table spoon (may use I teaspoon of dried ground ginger as well)

- Fresh minced garlic: 1 table spoon or 1 teaspoon of garlic powder.

- Worcestershire sauce: 1 table spoon

- Medium-large flank steak: 1  (around 1 1/2 pounds)

Method

1.  Place canola oil, chicken broth, honey, soy sauce, green onions, ginger, garlic powder, and Worcestershire sauce in a medium bowl. Mix with a whisk and keep aside.

2.  Remove any visible fat from the flank. Make slight cuts in the meat with serrated knife, scoring about 1/4-inch into the

meat in a crisscross fashion. Leave about an inch between cuts and do it both on the top and bottom of the flank.

3. Now lay the flank in a rectangular plastic container, add the marinade, and coat the steak well all over. Cover and marinate the flank steak all day or overnight, turning occasionally.

4. Set the grill and cook the flank for 10-15 minutes on each side or until cooked to your desired doneness. Use a carving knife to cut diagonally across the grain of the meat into slices of your desired thickness.

5. Serve with either sautéed vegetables or baked potatoes.

| Nutrition Facts |
| --- |
| Total calories: 350 |
| Fat: 56 g |
| Total Carbs: 18 g |
| Protein: 24 g |

## Day 6

### 11. Meal 1: Salmon with Apricot and Couscous

Time required: for Preparation: 20 minutes, cooking: 15 minutes

Skill level: advanced

You will need;

- Plain yogurt: 1/2 cup

- Scallions: 3 sliced, greens and whites separated

- Lemon juice: 2 tablespoons

- Fresh cilantro: 2 tablespoons chopped

- Ground cumin: 1/2 teaspoon

- Salt: as required

- Freshly ground pepper: 1/2 teaspoon

- Extra-virgin olive oil: 1 tablespoon

- Dried apricots: 1/4 cup chopped

- Minced fresh ginger: 1 tablespoon

- Whole-wheat couscous: 1 cup

- Salmon fillet: 1 pound (preferably wild Pacific, skinned and cut into 4 portions)

- Toasted cashews: 2 tablespoons, copped

Method

1. Set your oven to preheat at 475 F or medium-high.

2. Mix yogurt, scallion greens, lemon juice, cilantro, cumin, 1/4 teaspoon salt and 1/4 teaspoon pepper in a medium bowl. Keep aside.

3. Place a large saucepan over medium heat and put oil in it. Add apricots, ginger, the scallion whites and 1/4 teaspoon salt. Cook over medium heat while stirring until the apricots are soft. It usually takes 2 to 3 minutes. Add about 1 cup of water and bring to a boil over high heat. Mix in couscous. Remove from heat, cover and let stand until the liquid is absorbed, about 5 minutes. Fluff with a fork.

4. In the meantime, season salmon with about 1/4 teaspoon each salt and pepper. Oil the grill rack, place salmon and grill for about 3 minutes per side, until it is browned. You can also broil the salmon in the broiler.

5. Serve with the couscous, topped with the yogurt sauce and cashews.

| Nutrition Facts |
| --- |
| Total calories: 490 |
| Fat: 15 g |
| Total Carbs: 57 g |
| Protein: 35 g |

## 12. Meal 2: Spinach and Tomato Pasta

Time required: for Preparation: 20 minutes, cooking: 15 minutes

Skill level: easy

You will need;

- Cherry tomatoes: 1 cup cut into half

- Olive oil: 1 table spoon

- Spinach: 1 cup loosely packed fresh or frozen in bags

- Garlic: 1 tablespoon minced

- Whole wheat pasta: 2 cups cooked in small shapes like macaroni, rotelli, or small shells

- Parmesan cheese: 1/4 cup shredded

- Toasted pine nuts: 1 tablespoon

- Salt: as per taste

- Pepper: as per taste

Method

1. Pour olive oil in a medium size nonstick saucepan or skillet heated over medium-high heat. When the oil is nice and hot in about 30 seconds, add the tomatoes, spinach, and garlic and continue to sauté for a few minutes until spinach and tomatoes are soft and spinach is bright green  Sprinkle  some salt and pepper according to your taste.

2. Mix in the cooked pasta and continue to cook and stir

the mixture for a minute or two to heat up the pasta and blend the flavors.

3. Sprinkle parmesan cheese over the pasta and turn off the heat. Let the dish sit for a couple of minutes, garnish with pine nuts over the top, and serve!

| Nutrition Facts |
| --- |
| Total calories: 280 |
| Fat: 9 g |
| Total Carbs: 42 g |
| Protein: 11 g |

# Day 7

## 13. Meal 1: Beef & Cabbage Stir-Fry with Peanut Sauce

Time required: for Preparation: 40 minutes, cooking: 40 minutes

Skill level: Advanced

You will need;

- Smooth natural peanut butter: 1/4 cup

- Orange juice: 1/3 cup

- Low-sodium soy sauce: 3 tablespoons

- Rice vinegar: 1 tablespoon

- Sugar: 2 teaspoons

- Cooking oil, 2 tablespoons, divided

- Garlic: 4 cloves minced

- Sirloin steak: 1 pound trimmed and thinly sliced

- Savoy cabbage: 1 small head thinly sliced

- Carrots: 2 medium, grated

- Roasted peanuts: 1/ 4 cup chopped (optional)

Method

1. Blend peanut butter, orange juice, soy sauce, vinegar and sugar in a medium bowl with the help of whisk, until they become fluffy and you get a smooth mixture.

2. Add 1 tablespoon of oil in a wok or large skillet and heat over medium-high heat. Zap in garlic and cook, stirring, until fragrant for about 30 seconds. Put thinly sliced sirloin steak in the skillet and cook, stirring, until browned and barely pink in the middle. It will take about 2 to 4 minutes. Transfer it to a bowl.

3. Lower the heat and in the same skillet pour remaining 1 tablespoon of oil. Reduce heat to medium. Swirl in the remaining 2 teaspoons oil. Put cabbage and add 2 tablespoons of water; cook while stirring frequently until the cabbage begins to beginning to wilt, for about 3 to 5 minutes. Now also add carrots and some more water to avoid burning or sticking to the pan. Cook for 3 minutes more, till the carrots are tender.

4. Finally, transfer the steak back to the skillet. Remember to pour the accumulated juices in the bowl as well. Add the peanut sauce and toss to combine.

5. Serve with udon noodles, sprinkled with peanuts (if you are using them).

*Tip: Freeze the beef for at least 30 minutes before slicing. It will make easier to cut into very thin slices.*

| Nutrition Facts |
| --- |
| Total calories: 450 |
| Fat: 18 g |
| Total Carbs: 37 g |

| Protein: 31 g |
|---|

### 14. Meal 2: Broccoli cheesy soup

Time required: for Preparation: 20 minutes, cooking: 15 minutes

Skill level: Medium

You will need;

- Broccoli: 3 pounds( about 4 bunches)

- Green onion: 1/2 cup chopped

- Butter: 2 teaspoons

- Chicken broth: 2 cups

- Flour: 4 tablespoons

- Milk: 4 cups

- Swiss cheese: 3 cups, grated

Method

1.  Wash and drain the broccoli. Cut it into small pieces, removing the very thick bottom stems.

2.  Keep a medium pan with 2 cups water on high heat for boiling. Add broccoli when water starts boiling and cook only till it becomes tender. Over –cooking destroys the nutrients in vegetables. Drain the water, rinse with cold water and refrigerate.

3. In a large saucepan, sauté green onions for about two minutes in butter until tender.

4. Pour in the chicken broth and slowly add flour, stirring constantly to prevent lumps. Let the mixture come to slow boil on medium high heat. Once boiling, decrease heat to medium, and let it simmer for 5 minutes, stirring occasionally.

5. Add broccoli pieces to the broth and puree the mixture in an electric blender or food processor until smooth.

6. Again pour the soup to saucepan and cook over low heat. Add milk and Swiss cheese and simmer gently until cheese melts but be cautious that milk should not boil.

7. Serve hot and season with nutmeg, grated pepper, or grated cheddar cheese according to your liking.

| Nutrition Facts |
| --- |
| Total calories: 250 |
| Fat: 17 g |
| Total Carbs: 22 g |
| Protein: 10 g |

# 1 WEEK KETO MEAL PLAN

| Day | Breakfast | Lunch | Dinner | Net Carb | Total Calories |
|-----|-----------|-------|--------|----------|----------------|
| 1 | K-diet Breakfast Stack | Turkey and Vegetable Skillet | Baked Chicken Thighs with Cauliflower Mash | 5+3+4 = 12 | 680+674 +802= 2156 |
| 2 | Chicken and bacon patties | Apple Pork Chops with Roasted Broccoli | Beef Teriyaki with Sesame seeds & Kale | 3+6 +7= 16 | 370+717 +754= 1841 |
| 3 | Spanish Omelette with K-diet twist | Simple Egg Salad | Ground Beef Stir-Fry | 7+3 +9= 19 | 473+590 +620= 1683 |
| 4 | K- diet Apple Cinnamo n Muffins | Bacon and Avocado Salad | Spicy Chicken breasts with vegetables | 3+6 +9= 18 | 241+652 +576= 1469 |

| | | | | | |
|---|---|---|---|---|---|
| 5 | Italian Omelette | Chicken Cauliflower Salad | Quick Salmon Curry | 4+7+8 =19 | 555+ 371+ 909= 1835 |
| 6 | Baked Eggs in Avocados | Chicken Pepper Stir-Fry | K-diet Cottage Pie | 4+5+8 =17 | 500+ 595+ 684= 1779 |
| 7 | Keto Bacon Mini Frittata | Smoked Salmon and Ham Wraps with spinach | Creamy Tomato Basil Chicken "Pasta" | 3+2+ 11=16 | 460+ 382+ 633= 1475 |

# KETO RECIPES

## Day 1

### 15.Breakfast: K-diet Breakfast Stack

Time required: for Preparation: 15 minutes| Cooking: 15 minutes

Skill level: Medium

You will need;

- Bacon: 4 slices (112 g)

- Ground Beef; ¼ lbs. (110 g)

- Ground chicken1/4 lbs. (110 g)

- Egg: 1, whisked

- Italian seasoning; 2 teaspoons (2 g)

- Salt: 1 teaspoon (5 g)

- Black pepper: ¼ teaspoon approx. (1/2 g)

- Mushrooms: 2 large, stems removed

- Avocado: 1 thinly sliced

Method:

1. Take a large skillet, over medium-heat sauté bacon for about 5-6 minutes until crisp. Remove the bacon slices from skillet and place over a paper-lined plate to keep crisp. Save the bacon grease in the skillet.

2. Take another bowl, put ground chicken, ground beef

and mix with a whisked egg, Italian seasoning and salt. Make 4 thin patties out of the mixture.

3. Now, fry these patties over medium to high heat in the skillet with left over bacon grease. Cook for 3-4 minutes on each side till the patties are crisp and fully cooked. Take patties out of the skillet and set aside.

4. In the same skillet add mushrooms and cook them for 2-3 minutes until they're fully cooked from both sides. Take out the mushrooms and put aside.

5. To arrange the breakfast steak, first place each mushroom on a plate and stack with 2 patties, followed by 3 avocado slices and 2 slices of crisp fried bacon slices.

6. The K-diet breakfast steak is ready to be served. Place the remaining avocado slices in the plate when serving.

| Nutrition Facts |
| --- |
| Total calories: 680 |
| Fat: 54 g |
| Total Carbs: 13 g |
| Fiber: 8 g |
| Net Carbs: 5 g |
| Protein: 38 g |

### 16.Lunch: Turkey and Vegetable Skillet

Time required: for Preparation: 10 minutes | Cooking: 20 minutes

Skill level: Advanced

You will need;

● Coconut oil: ¼th cup (60 ml) for cooking

● Turkey breasts (either diced or ground turkey meat): 1 lb. (400 g)

● Diced bacon strips: 4 (112 g)

● Thinly sliced onion: 1 medium size (110 g),

● Chopped spinach: around 1 cup (30 g)

● Asparagus: 1 spears, chopped (22 g)

● Chopped fresh thyme: 1 tablespoon (3 g)

● Salt and pepper: according to your taste

Method

1. Melt the coconut oil over medium to high heat in a large skillet, put turkey and bacon and sauté them until meat is lightly browned. It will take approximately 5-7 minutes.

2. Now add onion, spinach, asparagus, and fresh thyme to the turkey and bacon mixture and cook for another 10 minutes so the meat is fully cooked and vegetables become soft.

3. Sprinkle pepper and salt according to your taste.

3. For serving, put the turkey and vegetable skillet in two plates and serve while hot.

| Nutrition Facts |
| --- |
| Total calories: 674 |
| Fat: 47 g |
| Total Carbs: 4 g <br> Fiber: 1 g <br> Net Carbs: 3 g |
| Protein: 61 g |

*Additional info; you can double the quantity of turkey, bacon and vegetables. After the mixture is prepared in skillet, save half for later use, (can be refrigerated for 3 days). For consuming, thoroughly heat the vegetable and turkey mixture over medium to high heat and add salt and pepper according to use.*

## 17.Dinner: Baked Chicken Thighs with Cauliflower Mash

Time required: for Preparation: 10 minutes | Cooking: 50 minutes

Skill level: medium

You will need:

For the baked chicken thighs -

● Olive oil; 2 Tablespoons of (30 ml), (plus some extra for the baking tray)

● Chicken thighs with skin; 6 (900 g)

● Salt: 1 tablespoon (15 g)

For the cauliflower mash -

● Cauliflower' small head (300 g), broken into small florets

● Coconut milk: ¼th cup (60 ml)

● Salt, to taste

Method:

For baking chicken thighs -

1. Preheat your oven to 450 F (230C). Take a rimmed baking tray and grease it with olive oil.

2. Put some salt on chicken thighs and rub well. Place these chicken thighs on the greased baking tray. Trickle one teaspoon of olive oil (5 ml) over each chicken thigh.

3. Lay the baking tray in the oven and bake for approximately 40 -50 or until the thighs are cooked through and the skin is crispy. You can check if the meat is fully cooked by inserting an instant-read meat thermometer. When internal temperature reaches 165 F (75 C), remove the baking tray from the oven and leave it for few minutes to cool down.

4. Divide the remaining chicken thighs between 2 plates and serve.

For making cauliflower mash -

1. First steam or boil cauliflower for 5-7 minutes, until the florets are soft. Drain the water well.

2. In a blender or food processor, blend cauliflower thoroughly with coconut milk. Add salt according to your taste. Season with salt, to taste. Refrigerate half of the cauliflower mash for

3. For serving divide the chicken thighs and cauliflower mash in two plates and serve hot.

| Nutrition Facts |
| --- |
| Total calories: 802 |
| Fat: 62 g |
| Total Carbs: 8 g |
| Fiber: 4 g |
| Net Carbs: 4 g |

**Protein: 51g**

*Additional info: You can prepare a large batch with double quantity and keep refrigerated for 3 days. Warm it thoroughly before use.*

## Day 2

### 18.Breakfast: Chicken and Bacon Patties

Time required: for Preparation: 10 minutes | Cooking: 20 minutes

Skill level: medium

You will need;

- Bacon: 2 slices (56 g)

- Chicken mince: 1 lb. (450 g)

- Egg: 1 medium, whisked

- Italian seasoning: 2 tablespoons (6 g)

- Garlic powder: 2 teaspoons (7 g)

- Onion powder: 2 teaspoons (5 g)

- Salt and pepper: according to your taste

Method:

1. Turn on your oven to preheat 425 F (220 C). Cover a rimmed baking tray with aluminum foil or parchment paper and set aside.

2. Take a small skillet and, sauté diced bacon for 2-5 minutes or until crispy. Take bacon out of the skillet with the help of a slotted spoon and place over the paper-towel lined plate to drain.

3. Now in a bowl, mix the cooked bacon with chicken mince, whisked egg, Italian seasoning, and garlic and onion

powder. Also add salt and pepper according to your taste.

4. Divide the mixture in to 12 parts to make 12 patties of approximately ½ inch thickness. Place these patties on the prior prepared baking tray.

5. Place the baking tray in the oven and bake for around 20 minutes until the patties are cooked thoroughly. You can check with an instant-read meat thermometer and the internal temperature of patties ideally would be around 170 F (76 C).

6. Let the patties sit for a while to cool down slightly. One person can consume 2-3 patties according to appetite, but remember to adjust accordingly your remaining intake during the day. Refrigerate leftovers in an airtight container, to be used later.

| Nutrition Facts |
|---|
| Total calories: 370 |
| Fat: 21 g |
| Total Carbs: 3 g |
| Fiber: 1 g |
| Sugar: 1 g |
| Net Carbs: 3 g |
| Protein: 40g |

### 19.Lunch: Apple Pork Chops with Roasted Broccoli

Time required: for Preparation: 10 minutes | Cooking: 20 minutes

Skill level: advanced

You will need;

For the pork chops -

- Pork chops: 2 (320 g)

- Ghee (clarified butter): 6 Tablespoons (90 ml)

- Applesauce: 2 tablespoons (30 ml)

- Mustard: 2 Tablespoon (30 ml)

- Salt and pepper, to taste

For the roasted broccoli -

- Broccoli: 1/2 head of (225 g), broken into small florets

- Olive oil: 1 Tablespoon (15 ml)

- Salt, to taste

Method:

To cook the pork chops -

1. Season the pork chops with salt and pepper.

2. In a large skillet, Place 4 Tablespoons (60 ml) of ghee and melt over high heat. With the help of the tongs place pork chops in the ghee on their sides, cook till the sides of the chops

are browned and crispy.

3. Now reduce the heat to medium level and place the chops flat in the skillet. Cook over on one side for about 3 minutes and then flip over to other side and cook for another 3-5 minutes until the chops are cooked to your liking. Check with an instant-read meat thermometer, recommended temperature for medium- rare is 145 F (63 C). Take out the pork chops from the skillet and let rest for 3 to 5 minutes.

4. Meanwhile, melt the remaining 2 table spoons of ghee over stovetop or in microwave and combine it with applesauce and mustard in a small bowl. Add salt and pepper, to taste

5. For serving, place the pork chops on 2 plates and serve with equal amounts of the prepared sauce.

For the roasted broccoli -

1. Preheat the oven to 450 F (230 C).

2. In a large bowl, mix the broccoli with the olive oil. Season it with salt. Place the broccoli in a single layer on a rimmed baking tray.

3. Place the baking tray in the oven and bake for 20 minutes until the broccoli is slightly crispy and cooked to your liking.

4. Place equal portions in two plates and serve with the pork chops.

**Nutrition Facts**

**Total calories: 717**

| | |
|---|---|
| Fat: 63 g | |
| Total Carbs: 10 g | |
| Fiber: 4 g | |
| Sugar: 4 g | |
| Net Carbs: 6 g | |
| Protein: 37  g | |

## 20. Dinner: Beef Teriyaki with Sesame seeds & Kale

Time required: for Preparation: 10 minutes | Cooking: 15 minutes

Skill level: medium

You will need;

• Wheat and soy -free sauce (tamari or coconut aminos): 2 tablespoons (30 ml)

• Applesauce: 1 tablespoon (15 ml)

• Garlic cloves: 2 (6 g), minced or finely diced

• Ginger: I table spoon (5 g), thinly sliced

• Beef steaks: 2 sliced (400 g)

• Sesame seeds: ½ tablespoon (7 g)

• Avocado oil: 2 tablespoons for cooking (30 ml)

• White button mushrooms: 10 (100 g), sliced

• Kale: 1 oz. (56 g), stems removed and chopped

• Sesame oil: 1 teaspoon (5ml) (or according to your taste)

• Salt and pepper: according to taste

Method:

1. Take a bowl, combine the wheat and soy free sauce, applesauce, finely diced garlic, and fresh ginger, and Wisk them well to form a marinade. Place the sliced beef steaks in the marinade and set aside.

2. In a nonstick skillet, dry roast the sesame seeds over high heat until golden.

Remove the sesame seeds from the skillet and keep aside.

3. Keep the flame high and in the same skillet put avocado oil, and add mushrooms. Cook mushrooms for 3-5 minutes until they are golden brown

4. Now add the beef steak with the marinade to the skillet and stir-fry until browned, in about 2 to 4 minutes.

5. Finally place sesame oil and kale in the skillet and cook for another few minutes until the kale is wilted and beef is cooked according to your taste. Season with salt and pepper, according to your taste.

6. To serve, place equal quantity of beef teriyaki in two plates. Garnish each plate with equal amounts of toasted sesame seeds and serve hot.

| Nutrition Facts |
| --- |
| Total calories: 754 |
| Fat: 62 g |
| Total Carbs: 10 g |
| Fiber: 3 g |
| Sugar: 2 g |
| Net Carbs: 7 g |
| Protein: 38 g |

## Day 3

### 21.Breakfast: Spanish Omelette with K-diet twist

Time required: for Preparation: 15 minutes | Cooking: 30 minutes

Skill level: easy

You will need;

● Olive oil: 2 tablespoons (30 ml), for cooking as well as for greasing the baking tray

● Cauliflower broken in to small florets: 1/4th cup (150 g)

● Bell peppers: 1 medium (120 g), thinly sliced

● Onion: 1 small (25 g), thinly sliced

● Eggs: 5, whisked

● Coconut cream: 2 tablespoons (30 ml) (you can get it from the top of a refrigerated tin of coconut milk)

● Fresh chopped parsley: 2 tablespoons (2 g)

● Avocado: ½, sliced (100 g)

● Salt and pepper, to taste

Method

1. First, set your oven to be pre-heated to 350 F (175 C). Grease a medium size baking dish with olive oil and keep aside.

2. In a pot, put water to boil and add salt. Add cauliflower to salted water, and boil for 2-3 minutes until somewhat tender. Drain cauliflower from water in a colander and set aside.

3. Next, put olive oil to a large skillet over medium-high heat. Add the bell pepper and onion to the skillet and sauté for about 6-8 minutes so that vegetables become soft. Add seasoning (salt and pepper) according to taste. Let the mixture to sit for few minutes to cool down slightly.

4. Take a large bowl, and mix the sautéed vegetables with the boiled cauliflower, add the whisked eggs, fresh parsley and coconut cream. Transfer the egg mixture into the greased baking dish. Place the dish in the pre-heated oven for approximately 20 minutes. Remember that eggs need to be cooked but still slightly soft.

5. Take the baking dish out of oven and let it cool a bit before serving.

6. Distribute the Omelette between 2 plates and top with equal amounts of sliced avocado.

| Nutrition Facts |
| --- |
| Total calories: 473 |
| Fat: 38 g |
| Total Carbs: 17 g |
| Fiber: 10 g |
| Sugar: 5 g |
| Net Carbs: 7 g |
| Protein: 19 g |

## 22. Lunch: Simple Egg Salad

Time required: for Preparation: 10 minutes | Cooking: 15 minutes

Skill level: easy

You will need;

● Medium sized eggs: 6

● Small onion: 1, thinly sliced (27 g),

● Regular mayonnaise; ¼th cup (60 ml)

● Mustard: 1 tablespoon (15 ml)

● Romaine lettuce: ½ head, finely chopped (100 g)

● Olive oil: 2 tablespoons (30 ml)

● Salt and black pepper: according to taste

Method:

1. Take a large pan, fill it with water to half of its capacity, place eggs and boil them for 3 minutes. After 3 minutes, remove from the flame and cover the pot with lid and let the eggs sit in water for almost 10 minutes. After wards drain water, remove egg shells and chop the eggs.

2. In a bowl, mix the chopped eggs and chopped onion with mustard and mayonnaise. Season with salt and pepper, according to your taste.

3. Take another bowl, place the romaine lettuce with the olive oil and toss it well.

4. For serving, place equal amounts of salad in two plates and top with equally divided egg mixture.

| Nutrition Facts |
| --- |
| Total calories: 590 |
| Fat: 57 g |
| Total Carbs: 4 g |
| Fiber: 2 g |
| Sugar: 2 g |
| Net Carbs: 2 g |
| Protein: 19 g |

## 23. Dinner: Ground Beef Stir-Fry

Time required: for Preparation: 10 minutes | Cooking: 15 minutes

Skill level: medium

You will need;

● Coconut oil: 2 Tablespoons (30 ml), for cooking

● Bell peppers 2 medium (240 g), cut in to slices (Julian slices)

● Cherry tomatoes: 10 (170 g), coarsely chopped

● Onion: ½ (55 g), thinly sliced

● Ground beef: 3/4 lbs. (338 g)

● Garlic: 2 cloves (6 g), crushed or finely diced

● Hot Sauce: 1 teaspoon of (5 ml) (the amount can be adjusted to taste or completely omitted))

● Fresh cilantro: 2 Tablespoons (2 g), chopped

● Salt and pepper, to taste

Method:

1. In a large skillet, melt the coconut oil over medium-high heat. Add the vegetables; bell peppers, tomatoes, and onion to the skillet and stir-fry for about 5 minutes, until they are slightly soft

2. Now, place the ground beef in the skillet and stir for 2-4 minutes until the meat is brown. Add garlic, hot sauce

(optional) and cilantro and continue stir frying till the ground beef is cooked to your taste.

3. Season with salt and pepper, to taste.

4. For serving, divide the ground brief in two equal portions and serve hot.

| Nutrition Facts |
| --- |
| Total calories: 620 |
| Fat: 50 g |
| Total Carbs: 13 g |
| Fiber: 4 g |
| Sugar: 6 g |
| Net Carbs: 9 g |
| Protein: 30 g |

## Day 4

### 24. Breakfast: K-diet Apple Cinnamon Muffins

Time required: for Preparation: 10 minutes | Cooking: 20 minutes

Skill level: easy

You will need;

- Almond flour: 3 cups (180 g)

- Ghee 1/2 cup (120 ml), plus some extra to grease the muffin pan)

- Applesauce: 1/4 cup (60 ml)

- Lemon juice: 1 teaspoon (5 ml)

- Eggs: 3 whisked

- Cinnamon powder: 3 Tablespoons (18 g)

- Nutmeg powder: 1 teaspoon (2 g)

- ground cloves: 1/4 teaspoon (1 g)

- Baking soda: 1 teaspoon (4 g)

- Stevia or low carb sweetener of choice, to taste

Method:

1. Preheat oven to 350 F (175 C). Take a 12-cup muffin pan, grease it with melted ghee or line with paper liners.

2. Mix all ingredients in a large bowl, whisk them until they make a smooth mixture. Pour the mixture into the

prepared muffin pan.

3. Put the baking pan in the pre-heated oven and bake for 18 to 20 minutes. You can check the muffins by inserting a tooth pick, when the toothpick comes out clean it means that the muffins are ready.

4. Take out the muffins from the oven and let them cool before serving. You can store the excess muffins in an air tight container.

| Nutrition Facts |
| --- |
| Total calories: 241 |
| Fat: 22 g |
| Total Carbs: 7g |
| Fiber: 4 g |
| Sugar: 2 g |
| Net Carbs: 3 g |
| Protein: 7 g |

## 25. Lunch: Bacon and Avocado Salad

Time required: for Preparation: 10 minutes | Cooking: 5 minutes

Skill level: easy

You will need;

For the salad -

• Bacon: 4 slices (112 g)

• Romaine lettuce 1 head (200 g)

• Cucumber: 1/2 (110 g)

• Onion:  1/4 medium (28 g)

• Avocado; large (200 g)

For the dressing -

• Mayonnaise: 1/2 cup (120 ml)

• Lemon juice: 2 Tablespoons of (30 ml)

• Mustard: 2 teaspoons (10 ml)

• Garlic powder: 2 teaspoons (7 g)

• Salt and pepper, to taste

Method:

1. Dice the bacon slices, chop romaine lettuce, make thin slices of cucumber and onion and avocado. Place the bacon to a large nonstick skillet over medium-high heat and sauté until crispy, for about 5 minutes.

2. Use a slotted spoon to remove bacon from the skillet and place on a paper towel-lined plate to drain and cool down slightly.

3. In a bowl, whisk together mayonnaise, lemon juice, mustard, and garlic powder. Season with salt and pepper, to taste.

4. Toss the dressing with the romaine lettuce leaves. Add the cucumber and onion to the bowl and toss to combine.

5. For serving, place equal portions of the salad on two plates, and place equal amounts of cooked bacon and sliced avocado over top.

| **Nutrition Facts** |
| --- |
| **Total calories: 652** |
| **Fat: 65 g** |
| **Total Carbs: 15 g** |
| **Fiber: 9 g** |
| **Sugar: 3 g** |
| **Net Carbs: 6 g** |
| **Protein: 10 g** |

## 26. Dinner: Spicy Chicken breast with vegetables

Time required: for Preparation: 10 minutes | Cooking: 5 minutes

Skill level: medium

You will need:

- Chicken breast: 1 (200 g)

- Garlic powder: 1 Tablespoon (10 g)

- Salt: 1 teaspoon (5 g)

- Onion powder: 1/2 Tablespoon (4 g)

- Chili powder: 1 teaspoon of (2 g) (or according to taste or completely remove if you don't like spicy food)

- Pepper: one pinch

- Avocado oil: 1 Tablespoon (15 ml)

- Avocado: 1 large (200 g)

- Bell pepper: 1 medium-size (120 g), chopped

- Cucumber: ½ (110 g), chopped

- Tomato: one medium (120 g)

- 1/4 medium (28 g), thinly sliced

- Olive oil: 2 Tablespoons (30 ml)

- Mustard: 1 teaspoon (5 ml)

Method:

1. Cut the chicken breast in small cubes. Prepare a marinade by adding garlic powder salt, onion powder, optional chili powder, and pepper. Mix the chicken in the marinade.

2. Pour the avocado oil in to a large skillet and place over medium-high heat. Add the marinated chicken to the skillet and sauté for around 5 minutes till the chicken is cooked well.

3. In the meanwhile, chop cucumber, bell pepper, tomato and make slices of onion and avocado. Mix all these ingredients with olive oil and mustard and also add the cooked chicken.

4. To serve, divide the spicy chicken between 2 plates and enjoy.

| Nutrition Facts |
| --- |
| Total calories: 576 |
| Fat: 46 g |
| Total Carbs: 18 g |
| Fiber: 9 g |
| Sugar: 5 g |
| Net Carbs: 9 g |
| Protein: 27 g |

## Day 5

### 27. Breakfast: Italian Omelette

Time required: for Preparation: 5minutes | Cooking: 5 minutes

Skill level: easy

You will need;

● Olive oil: 3 tablespoons (45 ml)

● Cherry tomatoes: 6-8 (60 g)

● Fresh basil: 2 tablespoon (6 g)

● Mozzarella slices 2 (50 g)

● Eggs; Medium 5

● Salt and pepper, to taste

Method;

1. Drizzle 2 1/2 tablespoon of the olive oil into an egg pan and place over medium heat.

2. In the meanwhile, chop the tomatoes, mozzarella cheese and basil leaves.

3. Break the eggs into a bowl, season with salt and pepper to taste, and whisk until they are frothy. Pour the egg mixture in to the heated pan and cook it for 1 minute over medium heat. Run spatula around the underside. Cook until the upper side and center look almost cooked.

4. Now place the tomatoes, mozzarella, and basil over

half of the Omelette, and fold the Omelette over the filling.

5. Turn off the heat but let the Omelette to sit in the pan for a minute. Pour the remaining ½ table spoon of olive oil over the Omelette.

6. Slide the Omelette gently on to the plate and divide in two equal parts for serving

| Nutrition Facts |
| --- |
| Total calories: 555 |
| Fat: 43 g |
| Total Carbs: 5 g |
| Fiber: 1g |
| Net Carbs: 4 g |
| Protein: 38 g |

## 28. Lunch: Chicken & cauliflower Salad

Time required: for Preparation: 15 minutes | Cooking: 10 minutes

Skill level: medium

You will need;

● Coconut oil: 1 Tablespoon (30 ml), for cooking

● Chicken breast:  1 (400 g)

● Cauliflower: ½ head (300 g)

● Cucumber: 1 small (120 g), diced

● Bell pepper: 1 small (80 g)

● Green onions: 2 (10 g)

● Fresh parsley 1/4 cup of (4 g),

● Olive oil: 1 Tablespoon (15 ml)

● Lemon juice ½ Tablespoon (7.5 ml) (or to taste)

● Garlic powder: 1 teaspoon of (3.5 g)

● Cumin powder:  1 teaspoon (2 g)

● Salt and pepper, to taste

Method:

1. First prepare all the ingredients; dice the chicken breast, cucumber and bell pepper. Chop green onions and fresh parsley. Put cauliflower in grinder / blender and process at low speed to get rice –like grains.

2. In a large skillet, melt the coconut oil over medium-high heat. Add the chicken to the skillet and sauté until fully cooked, about 8 to 10 minutes. Season with salt and pepper, to taste.

3. In another bowl, mix the cooked chicken, cauliflower, cucumber, bell pepper, green onions, and fresh parsley with the olive oil, lemon juice, garlic powder, and cumin powder. Season with additional salt and pepper, to taste.

4. Divide the salad between 2 bowls and serve.

| Nutrition Facts |
| --- |
| Total calories: 371 |
| Fat: 24 g |
| Total Carbs: 11 g |
| Fiber: 4 g |
| Sugar: 5 g |
| Net Carbs: 7 g |
| Protein: 27 g |

## 29. Dinner: Quick Salmon Curry

Time required: for Preparation: 15 minutes | Cooking: 10 minutes

Skills level: easy

You will need;

- Coconut oil: 2 Tablespoons (30 ml)

- Onion: 1/2 medium-size (55 g), thinly sliced

- Green beans: 7 oz. of (196 g), diced

- Chicken broth: 2 cups (480 ml)

- Salmon with skin: 1 lb. (450 g).the fish could be fresh or frozen, if frozen defrost first and then dice

- Curry powder: 1 1/2 Tablespoons (11 g)

- 1 teaspoon of garlic powder (3 g)

- Coconut cream: 1/2 cup of (120 ml) (from the top of a refrigerated tin of coconut milk)

- Fresh basil leaves (4 g), chopped for garnish

- Salt and pepper, to taste

Method

1. In a large pot, melt the coconut oil over medium-high heat. Add onion and sauté until translucent, for about 2 to 3 minutes.

2. Chop the green beans and add to the pot and cook for

few minutes until they are soft.

3. Now put the chicken broth in the saucepan and bring to a boil.

4. In the boiling broth add salmon, garlic powder and garlic powder and keep boiling for another one minute.

5. Decrease the heat to a simmer and add the coconut cream. Let the curry simmer at low heat, stirring carefully in between until the fish is fully cooked. Season with salt and pepper, to taste.

6. Serve the curry equally divided between 2 bowls and garnish with equal amounts of the fresh basil.

| Nutrition Facts |
| --- |
| Total calories: 909 |
| Fat: 67 g |
| Total Carbs: 15  g |
| Fiber: 7 g |
| Net Carbs: 8 g |
| Protein: 59 g |

## Day 6

### 30. Breakfast: Baked Eggs in Avocados

Time required: for Preparation: 10 minutes | Cooking: 15 minutes

Skill level: easy

You will need;

● Avocados:  2 large (400 g)

● Eggs: 4 medium

● Olive oil: 2 Tablespoons (30 ml)

● Salt and pepper, to taste

Method:

1. Set your oven to be pre-heated to 400 F (200 C).

2. Divide each avocado in to two halves cutting lengthwise. Remove the avocado seeds to have empty pits. Place each avocado half on a baking sheet.

3. Crack each egg into the avocado pit. Drizzle approximately 1 teaspoon of olive oil on to each avocado half.

4. Keep the baking sheet in the oven and bake for around 12 minutes.

6. When eggs are cooked, take out the baking dish, and season each avocado half with salt and pepper.

7. For serving, place 2 baked avocado halves on each plate and drizzle with the remaining olive oil.

| Nutrition Facts |
| --- |
| Total calories: 500 |
| Fat: 50 g |
| Total Carbs: 8 g |
| Fiber: 4 g |
| Net Carbs: 4 g |
| Protein: 17 g |

# 31.Lunch: Chicken Pepper Stir-Fry

Time required: for Preparation: 10 minutes | Cooking: 15 minutes

Skills level: easy

You will need;

- Coconut oil: 3 Tablespoons of (45 ml)

- Bell peppers: 2 medium (240 g)

- Chicken breasts: 2 (400 g)

- Gluten-free sauce (tamari or coconut aminos): 1 Tablespoon (15 ml)

- Chili powder (1 g) 1/4 teaspoon of (or to taste) (optional)

- Salt and pepper, to taste

Method:

1. Slice the chicken breasts, bell peppers.

2. Take a skillet; melt the coconut oil over medium-high heat. Add the bell peppers to the skillet and stir-fry until slightly softened, about 3 to 4 minutes.

3. Now put the chicken to the skillet and stir-fry until cooked through, about 8 to 10 minutes.

4. Add the gluten –free sauce and optional chili powder to the chicken and bell pepper mixture and cook for an additional 1 minute. Season with salt and pepper, to taste.

5. To serve, place equal amounts of stir fry chicken in two plates and enjoy.

| Nutrition Facts |
| --- |
| Total calories: 595 |
| Fat: 41 g |
| Total Carbs: 7 g |
| Fiber: 2 g |
| Sugar: 3 g |
| Net Carbs: 5 g |
| Protein: 48 g |

## 32. Dinner: K- Diet cottage pie

Time required: for Preparation: 15 minutes | Cooking: 45 minutes

Skills level: advanced

You will need;

● Cauliflower:  1/2 head (600 g), broken into small florets

● Ghee (clarified butter): 1 tablespoon (melted) (15 ml)

● Avocado oil: 2 Tablespoons (30 ml), for cooking and additional for greasing the baking dish.

● Onion:  1/2 medium (55 g),

● Ground beef: 1 lbs. (453 g)

● Carrot: 1 (100 g), grated

● Italian seasoning: 1 Tablespoon (6 g)

● Fresh parsley: 1 Tablespoon chopped (2 g)

● Salt and pepper, to taste

Method:

1. First prepare your ingredients; break cauliflower into small florets, grate carrot, chop onions and parsley. Preheat the oven to 350 F (175 C). Grease a baking dish (9-inch x 9-inch or 23 cm x 23 cm) with avocado oil and keep aside.

2. Boil water in a pan and boil cauliflower for about 5 to 10 minutes, until they are tender. Drain well. You can also steam then cauliflower florets.

3. In a blender or food processor, blend the cauliflower florets with melted ghee until you get a smooth mixture. Add salt according to your taste.

4. Now, warm the avocado oil in a skillet over medium-high heat. Add the onion to the skillet and sauté until translucent, about 4 to 5 minutes.

5. Place the ground beef and diced carrot to the skillet and cook until the ground beef is browned, for about 8 to 10 minutes. Add the Italian seasoning and fresh parsley to the skillet and sauté for an additional 1 to 2 minutes. Season with salt and pepper, to taste.

7. Spread the beef mixture in the bottom of the prepared baking dish. Top it with the cauliflower mash prepared earlier

8. Put the baking dish in the oven and bake for 30 minutes.

9. Remove the baking dish from the oven and let it cool slightly.

| Nutrition Facts |
| --- |
| Total calories: 684 |
| Fat: 57 g |
| Total Carbs: 13 g |
| Fiber: 5 g |
| Sugar: 6 g |

| Net Carbs: 8 g |
| --- |
| Protein: 32 g |

### 33. Breakfast: Bacon Mini Frittata

Time required: for Preparation: 10 minutes | Cooking: 30 minutes

Skills level: medium

You will need;

- Avocado oil, for greasing muffin pan

- Bacon: 2 slices (53 g), diced

- Asparagus: 4 spears of (64 g), finely chopped

- Onions: 2 Tablespoons chopped (30 g)

- Eggs: 4, whisked

- Coconut milk: 1/4 cup (60 ml)

- Salt and pepper, to taste

Method:

1. Preheat oven to 350 F (175 C). Grease a 6-cup muffin pan with avocado oil or line with paper liners.

2. Sauté the bacon over medium-high heat until crispy for about 4-5 minutes. Remove the bacon from the skillet with a slotted spoon and drain on a paper towel-lined plate.

3. In a small bowl, mix the cooked bacon, asparagus, and chopped onions with the eggs and coconut milk. Season with salt, to taste. Transfer equal amounts of the egg mixture into the prepared muffin pan.

4. Place the muffin pan in the oven and bake for 25 to 30 minutes until the eggs are set but still slightly soft. Let the frittata cool a little bit before serving.

5. You can make 12 Mini Frittata with doubling the amount of ingredients and keep the leftover muffins in refrigerator in an airtight container.

| Nutrition Facts |
|---|
| Total calories: 460 |
| Fat: 41 g |
| Total Carbs: 4 g |
| Fiber: 1g |
| Sugar: 2 g |
| Net Carbs: 3 g |
| Protein: 19 g |

## 34. Lunch: Smoked Salmon and Ham Wraps with spinach

Time required: for Preparation: 10 minutes | Cooking: 0 minutes

Skills level: advanced

You will need;

• Coconut cream: 2 Tablespoons (30 ml) (from the top of a refrigerated can of coconut milk)

• Ham slices: 8 (224 g)

• smoked salmon 6 oz. (168 g)

• Cucumber: 1/2 (110 g), thinly sliced

• Spinach: 4 cups of (120 g)

• Olive oil: 2 Tablespoons (30 ml)

• Salt and pepper, to taste

Method:

1. Place ham slices in a large plate, evenly equal amounts of coconut cream on each ham slice. Put equal amounts of smoked salmon and sliced cucumber on each ham slice. Roll each ham slice to create a wrap.

2. In a small bowl, toss the spinach with the olive oil. Season with salt and pepper, according to taste. Alternatively, you can also lightly blanch spinach in boiling water before mixing in olive oil.

3. Divide the spinach between 2 plates. Top each plate

with 4 ham wraps and serve.

| Nutrition Facts |
| --- |
| Total calories: 382 |
| Fat: 24 g |
| Total Carbs: 4 g |
| Fiber: 2 g |
| Sugar: 1 g |
| Net Carbs: 2 g |
| Protein: 38 g |

## 35. Dinner: Creamy Tomato Chicken "Keto Pasta"

Time required: for Preparation: 10 minutes | Cooking: 30 minutes

Skills level: medium

You will need;

- Coconut oil: 2 Tablespoons (30 ml)

- Chicken breasts: 2 (400 g)

- Diced tomatoes: 1 can of (14 oz. or 400 g)

- Coconut milk: 1/4 cup of (60 ml) (from the top of a refrigerated can of coconut milk)

- Fresh basil leaves: 1/2 cup (16 g)

- Garlic: 4 cloves (12 g)

- Zucchini: 1 (120 g)

- Salt and pepper, to taste

Method:

1. Start by preparing all ingredients; dice chicken breasts, drain the diced tomatoes form the can, chop garlic and fresh basil, make noodle-like long strands of zucchini with the help of a peeler (the zucchini pasta)

2. In a skillet, melt the coconut oil over medium-high heat. Add the chicken to the skillet and sauté until fully cooked, for about 8 to 10 minutes.

3. Add the diced tomatoes to the skillet and sauté until

soft, about 2 to 3 minutes.

4. Put in the coconut cream, fresh basil, and garlic to the skillet and cook until the sauce starts to thicken, for about 2 to 3 minutes. Season with salt and pepper, to taste.

5. For serving, place equal; quantity of zucchini "pasta" in 2 plates and top it with the chicken basil creamy sauce.

| Nutrition Facts |
| --- |
| Total calories: 633 |
| Fat: 40 g |
| Total Carbs: 15 g |
| Fiber: 4 g |
| Sugar: 6 g |
| Net Carbs: 11 g |
| Protein: 49 g |

## 36. Traditional Keto Coffee

Time required: for Preparation: 5minutes | Cooking: 0 minutes

Skills level: easy

You will need;

- Black coffee: 2 cups (480 ml)

- Ghee 2 Tablespoons of (30 ml)

- MCT oil: 1 teaspoon (5 ml) (or more, if desired)

Method

1. Mix the coffee, ghee, and MCT oil in a blender and blend until fully blended.

2. Divide the coffee between 2 mugs and serve.

| Nutrition Facts |
| --- |
| Total calories: 143 |
| Fat: 24 g |
| Total Carbs: 0 g |
| Fiber: 0 g |
| Sugar: 0g |
| Net Carbs: 0 g |

| Protein: 0 g |
|---|
| Protein: 0 g |

# Chapter Twelve

# **Conclusions**

For concluding this book, it seems very appropriate that we emphasize again that intermittent diet is not a one-size-fits-all kind of a solution; rather it's a framework, which can be tailored according to every individual's requirements, objectives and goals, body types and sensitivities.

It is expected that people will respond differently when they change the timings of their diet. There are many ways of doing intermittent fasting, but it's been found that 16/8 method is the most commonly used because of its easy to follow routine and great results. It gives you flexibility of choosing your eating and fasting window and you can reap benefits ranging from losing fat, gaining weight, hormonal balance, autophagy, mental clarity, clear skin, longevity and many more. Moreover, this eating pattern gives you a simpler life style, without unnecessarily spending too much time in preparing and eating meals which your body does not actually require.

With all the information and guidance along with meal plans and recipes you have gained through this book, it's time for you to start your journey of intermittent fasting. First you have to decide about your eating and fasting period, which will depend on your lifestyle and meal schedules. So, once you figure out; when to eat, you can move on to more difficult part; what to eat. Get going and track your progress by stepping on scale, taking photos, checking fitting of your clothes, but, more importantly listen to your body. If you are feeling good about it then keep going.

In this journey, the mileage will vary between people but it's important that you are covering ground and moving forward. You will have your desired results in due time.

*Emily Lewis*

# THANK YOU
# FOR READING!

Made in the USA
Columbia, SC
26 January 2020